Natural PHARMACIST™

‖‖‖‖‖‖‖‖‖‖‖‖‖‖‖‖‖‖‖‖
W9-BNO-650

Inside—Find the Answers to These Questions and More

☑ What are the symptoms of a migraine headache? (See page 9.)

☑ What exactly *is* feverfew and how well does it help migraines? (See page 1.)

☑ What type of feverfew is best? (See page 95.)

☑ How much feverfew should I take? (See page 95.)

☑ Are there side effects? (See page 102.)

☑ Who should avoid feverfew? (See page 100.)

☑ What are the differences between migraine relief medications and migraine prevention medications? (See page 56.)

☑ Can the mineral magnesium help migraines? (See page 120.)

☑ What is 5-HTP, and why is it sometimes recommended for migraines? (See page 125.)

☑ Can acupuncture produce long-lasting relief for migraines? (See page 132.)

THE NATURAL PHARMACIST Library

Arthritis

Diabetes

Echinacea and Immunity

Feverfew and Migraines

Garlic and Cholesterol

Ginkgo and Memory

Heart Disease Prevention

Herbs

Illnesses and Their Natural Remedies

Kava and Anxiety

Menopause

PMS

Reducing Cancer Risk

Saw Palmetto and the Prostate

St. John's Wort and Depression

Vitamins and Supplements

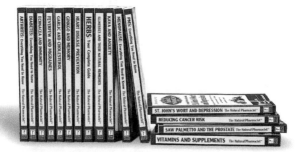

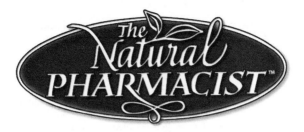

Everything You Need to Know About

Feverfew and Migraines

David Baronov, Ph.D.

Series Editors

Steven Bratman, M.D.

David Kroll, Ph.D.

A DIVISION OF PRIMA PUBLISHING

Visit us online at www.thenaturalpharmacist.com

Warning—Disclaimer

This book is not intended to provide medical advice and is sold with the understanding that the publisher and the author are not liable for the misconception or misuse of information provided. The author and Prima Publishing shall have neither liability nor responsibility to any person or entity with respect to any loss, damage, or injury caused or alleged to be caused directly or indirectly by the information contained in this book or the use of any products mentioned. Readers should not use any of the products discussed in this book without the advice of a medical professional.

The Food and Drug Administration has not approved the use of any of the natural treatments discussed in this book. This book, and the information contained herein, has not been approved by the Food and Drug Administration.

Pseudonyms are used throughout to protect the privacy of the individuals involved.

PRIMA HEALTH and colophon are trademarks of Prima Communications, Inc.

THE NATURAL PHARMACIST™ is a trademark of Prima Communications, Inc.

All products mentioned in this book are trademarks of their respective companies.

Interior illustrations by Lisa Cooper and Helene D. Stevens.

Illustrations © 1999 Prima Publishing. All rights reserved.

Library of Congress Cataloging-in-Publication Data

Baronov, David.
    The natural pharmacist guide to feverfew and migraines / David Baronov.
        p.   cm—(The natural pharmacist)
    Includes bibliographical references and index.
    ISBN 0-7615-1753-7
    1. Migraine—Alternative treatment.   2. Feverfew—Therapeutic use.
    I. Title. II. Series.
RC392.B37   1998
616.8'5706—dc21
                                        98-50346
                                          CIP

99 00 01 02 HH 10 9 8 7 6 5 4 3 2 1
Printed in the United States of America

Visit us online at www.thenaturalpharmacist.com

Contents

What Makes This Book Different?

The interest in natural medicine has never been greater. According to the National Association of Chain Drug Stores, 65 million Americans are using natural supplements, and the number is growing! Yet, it is hard for the consumer to find trustworthy sources for balanced information about this emerging field. Why? Frankly, natural medicine has had a checkered history. From snake oil potions sold at the turn of the century to those books, magazines, and product catalogs that hype miracle cures today, this is a field where exaggerated claims have been the norm. Proponents of natural medicine have tended to abuse science, treating it more as a marketing tool than a means of discovering the truth.

But there is truth to be found. Studies of vitamins, minerals, and other food supplements have been with us since these nutritional substances were first discovered, and the level and quality of this science has grown dramatically in the last 20 years. Herbal medicine has been neglected in the United States, but in Europe, this, the oldest of all healing arts, has been the subject of tremendous and ongoing scientific interest.

At present, for a number of herbs and supplements, it is possible to give reasonably scientific answers to the questions: How well does this work? How safe is it? What types of conditions is it best used for?

THE NATURAL PHARMACIST series is designed to cut through the hype and tell you what we know and what we don't know about popular natural treatments. These books are more conservative than any others available, more honest about the weaknesses of natural approaches, more fair in their comparisons of natural and conventional treatments. You won't find any miracle cures here; but you will discover useful options that can help you become healthier.

Why Choose Natural Treatments?

Although the science behind natural medicine continues to grow, this is still a much less scientifically validated field than conventional medicine. You might ask, "Why should I resort to an herb that is only partly proven, when I could take a drug with solid science behind it?" There are at least three good reasons to consider natural alternatives.

First, some herbs and supplements offer benefits that are not matched by any conventional drug. Vitamin E is a good example. It appears to help prevent prostate cancer, a benefit that no standard medication can claim. Also, vitamin E almost certainly helps prevent heart disease. While there are standard drugs that also prevent heart disease, vitamin E works differently and may be able to complement many of the other approaches.

Another example is the herb milk thistle. Studies strongly suggest that this herb can protect the liver from injury. There is no pill or tablet your doctor can prescribe to do the same.

Even if the science behind some of these treatments is less than perfect, when the risks are low and the possible benefit high, a treatment may be worth trying. It is a little-known fact that for many conventional treatments the science is less than perfect as well, and physicians must balance uncertain benefits against incompletely understood risks.

A second reason to consider natural therapies is that some may offer benefits comparable to those of drugs with fewer side effects. The herb St. John's wort is a good example. Reasonably strong scientific evidence suggests that this herb is an effective treatment for mild to moderate depression, while producing fewer side effects on average than conventional medications. Saw palmetto for benign enlargement of the prostate, ginkgo for relieving symptoms and perhaps slowing the progression of Alzheimer's disease, and glucosamine for osteoarthritis are other examples. This is not to say that herbs and supplements are completely harmless—they're not—but for most the level of risk is quite low.

Finally, there is a philosophical point to consider. For many people, it "feels" better to use a treatment that comes from nature instead of from a laboratory. Just as you might rather wear all-cotton clothing than polyester, or look at a mountain landscape rather than the skyscrapers of a downtown city, natural treatments may simply feel more compatible with your view of life. We can quibble endlessly about just what "natural" means and whether a certain treatment is "actually" natural or not, but such arguments are beside the point. The difference is in the feeling, and feelings matter. In fact, having a good feeling about taking an herb may lead you to use it more consistently than you would a prescription drug.

Of course, at times synthetic drugs may be necessary and even lifesaving. But on many other occasions it may be quite reasonable to turn to an herb or supplement instead of a drug.

To make good decisions you need good information. Unfortunately, while hundreds of books on alternative medicine are published every year, many are highly misleading. The phrase "studies prove" is often used when the studies in question are so small or so badly conducted that they prove nothing at all. You may even find that the "data" from other books comes from studies with petri dishes and not real people!

You can't even assume that books written by well-known authors are scientifically sound. Many of these authors rely on secondary writers, leading to a game of "telephone" where misconceptions are passed around from book to book. And there's a strong tendency to exaggerate the power of natural remedies, whitewashing them with selective reporting.

THE NATURAL PHARMACIST series gives you the balanced information you need to make informed decisions about your health needs. Setting a new, high standard of accuracy and objectivity, these books take a realistic look at the herbs and supplements you read about in the news. You will encounter both favorable and unfavorable studies in these pages and will learn about both the benefits and the risks of natural treatments.

THE NATURAL PHARMACIST series is the source you can trust.

Steven Bratman, M.D.
David Kroll, Ph.D.

nated in the Balkans, but no one knows its exact place of origin. Today the plant is found throughout Europe, and in North America from Quebec to Maryland and as far west as Ohio.

Like many medicinal herbs, feverfew is a weed. It thrives in diverse conditions but is most at home in semi-shaded, well-drained soil. It can grow to a height of 2 feet, rising along a furrowed, hairy stem. The flowers of the feverfew plant look a bit like daisies, with small, flat, yellow heads each ringed by 10 to 20 white-toothed petals. In fact, feverfew belongs to the daisy family *(Asteraceae)*. The plant's delicate, feathery green leaves grow to be about 4.5 inches long and 2 inches wide (see figure 1).

Feverfew *(Tanacetum parthenium)* is a rather unassuming perennial plant noted for its light green leaves, which emit a strong, bitter scent.

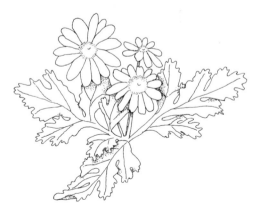

Figure 1. *Feverfew*

What's in a Name?

You may read in popular articles that feverfew lowers fevers. However, the name "feverfew" does not appear to be a reference to fevers at all. According to herbalist Michael Castleman, it is a corruption of the word "featherfoil," referring to the shape of the leaves.[1] "Featherfoil" became "featherfew," and then "feverfew." Interestingly, this transformation of the name had the ironic consequence of reducing the herb's popularity.

You might say that feverfew was an early victim of unintentional false advertising. Here's what happened: Professional herbalists did not know the linguistic origin of the name. They quite naturally assumed that feverfew must reduce fevers, and they tried to use it for this purpose. Unfortunately, it wasn't effective. After trying it unsuccessfully for a century or so, they decided the herb was no good and stopped using it entirely.

Fortunately, the older tradition of using feverfew for migraine headaches remained alive as a folk remedy, allowing it to resurface in the twentieth century.

Identifying feverfew in the wild can be challenging. Feverfew plants are similar to chrysanthemums, but smaller. They can easily be confused with chamomile, although the feverfew plant has an upright stem in contrast to the slightly bent stem of chamomile. The difficulty of identifying feverfew has proved troublesome. Herbal suppliers have been known to mistakenly ship bushels of German chamomile (*Matricaria recutita*) or German tansy (*Tanacetum vulgare*) in lieu of feverfew.

Why Is It Called Feverfew?

Over the centuries, feverfew has acquired an impressive list of popular names, including featherfoil, flirtwort, midsummer daisy, nosebleed, mutterkraut, and bachelor's button (not to be confused with the common blue or pink garden flower called "bachelor's button").

The Greeks called it *parthenion*, probably from the herb's use as a birthing medication. Variations of the Greek word *partheno* appear in many words associated with birth, such as *postpartum* and *parthenogenesis*.

The common English name "feverfew" is a variation on the medieval "featherfoil," referring to the herb's feathery leaves.[2] Over the years, "featherfoil" became "featherfew" and eventually "feverfew." See sidebar, What's in a Name?, for the story of how this progression of names led to a misunderstanding that persists to the present day.

What Is in Feverfew?

Like all herbs, feverfew is made up of hundreds of chemicals in varying concentrations. There are 15 to 20 important organic chemicals in feverfew, and no one really knows which of these chemicals are responsible for feverfew's medicinal effect. Until recently, most people thought that a single chemical, *parthenolide,* was the active ingredient in feverfew. Recent clinical studies, however, have cast serious doubt on this theory. This matter will be discussed in greater detail in chapter 5.

Like all herbs, feverfew is made up of hundreds of chemicals in varying concentrations.

The major chemical constituent of feverfew is a group of chemicals called *sesquiterpene lactones*. These chemicals are used by plants and humans alike to make such diverse compounds as plant growth hormones, cholesterol, and steroid hormones like estrogen and testosterone. The feverfew plant uses such building blocks instead to make parthenolide, which belongs to this group and accounts for 85% of total sesquiterpene lactone content. In addition to the sesquiterpene lactones, feverfew's major chemical constituents include essential oils, bitter resin, inulin (in the root), and pyrethrin.

What Was Feverfew Used for Historically?

Steven Foster, the eminent American herbalist, notes that the first recorded use of feverfew was by Dioscorides, a first-century Greek physician who prescribed it for a number of medicinal purposes. In particular, Dioscorides was said to have used feverfew for women in various stages of giving birth, and to treat menstrual conditions. Over the centuries, feverfew has been used for a perplexing array of maladies: fevers, headaches, vertigo, menstruation, morning sickness, labor, toothaches, stomachaches, kidney pain, hangovers, and insect bites.

Sir John Hill was an influential eighteenth-century English physician. In his description of feverfew in 1772, he wrote that "in the worst headaches, this herb exceeds whatever else is known." Indeed, across much of Europe, feverfew came to be known as the "aspirin of the eighteenth century." Nicholas Culpepper, a sixteenth-century astronomer and herbalist, wrote glowingly of feverfew's myriad of medical applications, from headache relief to the removal of freckles:

> *It is very effectual for all pains in the head coming of a cold cause, the herb being bruised and applied to*

*the crown of the head; as also for the vertigo. The
decoction, drunk warm, and the herb bruised with a
few corns of bay-salt, and applied to the wrists before the coming on of ague fits, do take them away.
The distilled water taketh away freckles and other
spots and deformities of the face. The herb bruised
and heated on a tile, with some wine to moisten it,
or fried with a little wine and oil, and applied warm
outwardly to the places, removes wind and colic
in the lower part of the belly. It is an especial
remedy against opium taken too liberally.*

As we've already seen, such unfounded claims—as
well as the false belief that feverfew could prevent or treat
fevers—ultimately led to a decline in feverfew's popularity. Subsequent herbalists spoke of feverfew as an ineffective treatment. As late as 1983, the British Herbal
Medicine Association failed to include feverfew in its
British Herbal Pharmacopoeia. It wasn't until the incident
with the young coal miner that medical professionals again
became interested in feverfew. Today, feverfew is generally used only for migraine headaches.

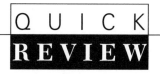

QUICK
REVIEW

- Feverfew *(Tanacetum parthenium)* has been known as a treatment for headaches since at least the eighteenth century.
- Feverfew is a perennial plant belonging to the daisy *(Aster-aceae)* family. Like many medicinal herbs, it is a weed that thrives in diverse conditions.

- Feverfew can be found throughout Europe and in eastern North America.

- The name "feverfew" is derived from the word "featherfoil," which refers to the plant's feathery, light green leaves.

- Feverfew is not effective for the treatment of fevers, as its name would suggest.

- Feverfew was rediscovered by European medicine in the 1970s, after a coal miner offered it as a folk treatment for the wife of the chief medical officer of the British National Coal Board. Since then, it has become a leading treatment for migraine headaches in the United Kingdom. As we will see in chapter 5, preliminary research suggests that this use is justified. More recently, it has begun to be prescribed by North American doctors and herbalists.

- Until recently, scientists thought that parthenolide was the active ingredient responsible for feverfew's effect of relieving migraine headaches. However, recent research has cast doubt on this explanation. We don't really know what the active chemical or chemicals in feverfew may be.

The Symptoms of a Migraine

An estimated 25 million Americans suffer from migraine headaches, and more than 4 million suffer from one migraine headache a week. For reasons that are not entirely clear, three out of every four people with migraines are women (see figure 2).

A migraine is a particular type of headache, although the symptoms vary widely among individuals with migraines. As we will see in chapter 4, we aren't sure exactly what causes migraine headaches. We do know that they all involve certain characteristic changes in the blood vessels, electrical activity, and chemistry of the brain.

The pain of migraine headaches varies considerably. Some people have migraines that are mild and infrequent. For many people, however, migraines are extremely painful and debilitating.

This chapter describes the symptoms of migraine headaches. Chapter 9 will help you determine whether your headache is a migraine or some other type of headache. If you do suffer from migraines, this book will

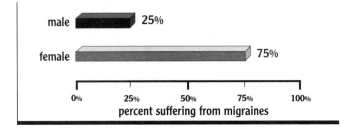

Figure 2. *More women than men suffer from migraines*

give you information about feverfew and other treatments that might help.

As you read this chapter, keep in mind that migraine headaches can be difficult to identify. Most migraine headaches do not conform to the classic migraine pattern in all respects, and symptoms can vary from the subtle to the overwhelming. Even doctors can fail to identify migraine headaches. A team of neurologists were recently quoted in the *British Journal of Medicine* as saying: "Migraine is common; if it is not diagnosed regularly in general practice it is being missed."[1]

Diagnosing Migraine Headaches

As we will see in chapter 9, diagnosing headaches isn't a straightforward process. A doctor can test you for diabetes or pneumonia, but no test can objectively tell you or your doctor that you suffer from migraines.

You don't need anyone to tell you that you have a headache, of course, but you do need your doctor's help to determine what type of headache it is, what its cause might be, and how to treat it. Your doctor, in turn, relies on you for information about the pain you feel.

How Many Men and Women Have Migraines?

A recent survey of over 20,000 people in the United States suggests that 17.6% of females and 5.7% of males have one or more migraines per year. According to the same survey, 3.4 million women and 1.1 million men have more than one severe headache per month.[2]

Because the diagnosis of a migraine is based on your own description of the pain, it's very important that you communicate well with your doctor. This chapter will help you learn how to describe your headaches clearly and, ideally, avoid misdiagnosis.

All headaches are categorized according to the nature of the pain they inflict. The nature of the pain is described in terms of five factors:

You don't need anyone to tell you that you have a headache, of course, but you do need your doctor's help to determine what type of headache it is.

1. The *intensity* of your headache—the relative degree of your discomfort or pain.
2. The *duration* of your headache—how long it lasts.
3. The *frequency* of your headaches—how often they occur.
4. The *location* of your headache— the specific area of your head that hurts.

Evaluating Your Own Headache

Under each category, choose the listed item that best describes your headache. This should help you describe your headaches more effectively to your doctor.

Intensity of pain:

- mild
- moderate
- severe
- debilitating

Duration of headache:

- lasting several minutes
- lasting an hour or longer
- lasting a day or longer
- lasting several days
- lasting a week or more

5. The *type* of pain associated with your headache—for example, dull and constant versus sharp and stabbing.

Intensity of Pain

As we'll see in this chapter, migraine headaches can be extremely intense. The intensity of the pain you feel can be mild, moderate, severe, or debilitating. Mild pain is

Frequency of headaches:

- occurring once a month
- occurring once every two weeks
- occurring once a week
- occurring once a day
- occurring several times a day

Location of pain:

- back of head (occipital)
- front of head (frontal)
- sides of head (temporal)
- top of head (vertex)
- area above or behind eyeball (sinus region)
- upper/lower jaw area (mandible)

Type of pain:

- varying (see text for different types and explain to your doctor the type that best describes your headache)

uncomfortable, but it doesn't disrupt your normal daily routine. Moderate pain interferes with one or more of your daily activities but isn't severe enough to be disruptive. For example, a moderately painful headache will make you decide to skip your workout but isn't too severe for you to drive yourself home. Further up the continuum is severe pain. A severe headache is painful enough to make it dangerous to drive and difficult or impossible to do anything except rest quietly. At its most intense, pain becomes completely debilitating.

These measures of intensity are very imprecise. People vary in their tolerance of pain, and also in their willingness to acknowledge it. For example, Ed is a retired longshoreman. To his way of thinking, acknowledging pain is not very manly, and once he actually went a whole day with a broken foot without admitting he had a problem. On the other hand, his friend Brad is so oversensitive that a paper cut can put him out of commission for a couple of hours. Between these two extremes there is a wide spectrum of sensitivity.

A severe headache is painful enough to make it dangerous to drive and difficult or impossible to do anything except rest quietly.

There is no way to know whether one person's headache is worse than another's. But you can rate the extent to which your headaches disrupt your everyday activities, and use the scale of intensity to learn more about your headaches' patterns. Are they always equally intense, or do they vary from mild to severe? These are important questions for you and your doctor to address.

Duration of Headache

The duration of your headaches refers to how long they last. The duration of migraines varies widely; for example, a headache can last from as little as 15 minutes to as long as a week or more. Longer duration does not necessarily mean a more serious condition. Some types of headaches, such as cluster headaches, are characterized by relatively brief bouts of debilitating pain. Other headaches, such as tension headaches, are characterized by longer periods of mild to moderate pain.

Frequency of Headaches

The frequency of your headaches refers to how often they occur. The frequency of migraines also varies. For example, headaches can occur very rarely (once every few years) or as often as once or twice a week. As a rule, migraines do not occur on a daily basis. Because the frequency of migraines is often similar to that of other headaches, frequency alone is not a good way to diagnose your headache.

Location of Pain

The location of your pain is another important clue to determine the type of headache you have. For example, a person with a tension headache generally experiences the pain as a bandlike pressure around the circumference of the head, and a sinus headache is usually felt on the forehead or face. But nearly 60% of the time, migraine headaches occur on just one side of the head and are centered above or behind one eye. The particular side of the headache often changes from one headache episode to the next. During a migraine attack, the pain can migrate from the original area of pain and even travel down the neck and into the shoulder. Frequently, the pain spreads during the course of the migraine, often until it covers the entire head.

Nearly 60% of the time, migraine headaches occur on just one side of the head and are centered above or behind one eye.

Doctors refer to seven specific regions of the head (see figure 3). When you describe your headache to your physician, you should make it clear which of these region(s) your pain is located in:

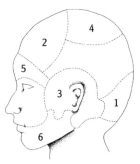

Figure 3. *The six regions of the head where migraine pain is most frequently experienced*

1. The back of the head (occipital).
2. The front of the head (frontal area).
3. The sides of the head (temporal).
4. The top of the head (vertex).
5. The area between and above the eyebrows and behind the cheekbones (sinus region).
6. The upper/lower jaw area (mandible).

Of course, pain can occur in more than one of these regions at a time. Location may help you determine which type of headache you have, but it's not a reliable indicator of the *cause* of your headache. (See chapter 3 for a discussion of what causes a migraine headache.)

Type of Pain

Arguably, the type of pain is the most subjective of these four factors. How can we really communicate to another person what the pain in our head feels like?

Doctors find it useful to rely on certain vivid terms that help distinguish one kind of pain from another. Migraine pain is usually described as pounding, pulsating, or throbbing. The throbbing of a migraine headache often

The Pain of a Migraine

Cassandra always knew when a migraine was coming. She might wake up in the middle of the night in her dark bedroom and find that her eyes were blinking, as if to ward off a bright light. "When I have a migraine," she said, "light *hurts*. I can't bear to have the blinds open."

The sharp pain first appeared in a spot just above her right eyebrow. The pain was invariably intense and throbbing, Cassandra said, "as if a knife was plunged into just that spot." Then the pain slowly spread across her forehead, until it felt like a tight band. At this point, Cassandra would become severely nauseated and begin to vomit. "It feels," she said, "like I'm barfing up my *feet*."

Between the nausea and the pain, Cassandra felt completely incapacitated. She couldn't lift her head, and the pain left her little room for thought. Cassandra's headaches always lasted about 24 hours. During a headache she would take naps and wake to find the pain was still there, until finally the headache wound down. The day after a migraine, Cassandra felt weak and drained, as if she had the flu.

feels as if it is following the rhythm of your heartbeat. As we will see in chapter 3, this rhythmic throbbing is an important clue to the physiological mechanisms behind migraine headaches. The pain is also described as shooting or burning, sharp or dull, and hot or without noticeable temperature. Pain can be heavy and diffused, or sharply localized. It can press or squeeze. You can also use metaphors to describe the pain. "I feel as if an ice pick

Barbara's and Tim's Stories

Barbara had all the symptoms of a classic migraine. She could always tell when a headache was coming: She felt dizzy and confused, and she saw geometric shapes that remained whether she opened her eyes or kept them shut. Soon after the dizzy spell, the pain would begin: a pounding sensation above or behind one eye.

Once a headache began, Barbara knew it would last for several hours. Each headache seemed to have a distinct beginning, middle, and end. At its peak, the headache was excruciatingly painful. In addition to the head pain, Barbara always felt severely nauseated, and she couldn't stand strong smells or any amount of light. Gradually, after hours of agony,

is buried in my temple," you might say; or, "I feel as if I'm being hit with a hammer." Although the type of pain doesn't automatically tell you what kind of headache you have, it's a clue—and, as we will see later in this chapter, the type of pain is a particularly important piece of information for screening you for any serious medical conditions.

Four out of five migraines *don't* fit the classic pattern.

The sidebar Barbara's and Tim's Stories shows the paradoxical nature of migraine headaches. About 20% of migraines fit the classic pattern of Barbara's experience. In other words, four out of five migraines *don't* fit the classic pattern. A classic migraine is very easy to identify, as we will she would begin to feel the headache slip away, until finally she was free of pain. After a migraine, she felt a bit weak and delicate for a few hours.

Tim had a very different problem: From time to time he would suddenly develop a deep pounding pain in his neck. These episodes, which lasted a few hours at a time, were extremely painful, but neither he nor his doctor could find the cause. His neck didn't seem to be injured or to have any skeletal problems. Massage didn't help. Sometimes the neck pain was accompanied by very mild nausea, but Tim didn't have any other symptoms.

Like Barbara, Tim was experiencing migraines.

see later in this chapter. But for the vast majority of people with migraines, diagnosis can be more difficult. In fact, sometimes a doctor will prescribe a migraine medication for a hard-to-identify headache. If the medication helps, then the headache is presumed to have been a migraine.

Migraine Symptoms Other Than Head Pain

Aside from head pain, many other physical symptoms often accompany migraine headaches. Again, not all people who experience migraines also experience these symptoms, but they are fairly common. These other symptoms include nausea and vomiting; fever and chills; and a heightened sensitivity to light, sound, and odors. Some people with migraines also experience diarrhea, lightheadedness, tenderness of the scalp, and facial swelling, while others experience nasal congestion and a pressure around the sinuses. Physical activity tends to heighten the pain of these symptoms, as well as of the headache itself.

Severe nausea is a characteristic symptom of migraine. It can be particularly troublesome, depending on how severe it is and whether it leads to actual vomiting. Excessive vomiting can prevent oral medications from being effectively absorbed.

Following a migraine attack, there are further symptoms you may experience. Typically, you may feel irritable and listless, with impaired concentration once the headache has lifted.

> **Severe nausea is a characteristic symptom of a migraine. It can be particularly troublesome, depending on how severe it is and whether it leads to actual vomiting.**

Common Migraine Versus Classic Migraine

A *classic* migraine, as we saw above in Barbara's story, is preceded by a set of neurological symptoms, such as dizziness or visual symptoms. This set of symptoms is called an *aura.* No one knows exactly why the aura occurs or what it is, but we can assume that it is caused by both chemical and electrical changes in the brain, and possibly a reduction in the flow of blood to the brain. (See chapter 3 for a discussion of the cause of migraine headaches.) Approximately one in five people who experience migraines has classic migraines preceded by an aura.

The aura occurs 10 to 30 minutes before the beginning of a migraine attack, and it may return at various times throughout the headache. Many people describe the aura as a peculiar visual distortion. A castlelike structure slowly passes across the field of vision, blocking out objects and confusing the person experiencing the migraine, who may become dizzy and disoriented throughout this period. This can be an extremely disturbing and scary experience. Typically, an aura includes both visual and other sensory symptoms.

One common visual symptom is the appearance of a bright shape passing across the field of vision, blocking the sight in one eye and remaining visible even when the eyes are closed. Some people temporarily lose their sight altogether. Another visual symptom that frequently comes during the aura is a series of wavy lines or geometric patterns appearing before the eyes. Flashing lights and colors may also appear.

One visual symptom that frequently comes during the aura is a series of wavy lines or geometric patterns appearing before the eyes.

The partial loss of sight during an aura is referred to as *scotoma.* The phenomenon of flashing lights is known as *photopsia.* Further symptoms associated with an aura include a difficulty with speech, weakness in an arm or leg, a tingling of the face or hands, weakness or heaviness in the limbs, and a sense of confusion.

In contrast to a classic migraine, a *common* migraine is not preceded by an aura. The common migraine is well named, since the vast majority of migraine headaches belong in this category. However, many people with common migraines do experience some symptoms just before a migraine attack. The period before the onset of the headache pain is known as the *prodrome*. The prodrome of a common migraine can include symptoms such as mood changes, fatigue, and increased urination.[3] These symptoms are generally less well defined than the symptoms of an aura. Migraines may occur at any time of day or night but will often strike when you are just waking up in the morning.

Are Migraines Hereditary?

A tendency to migraines may be genetic. Between 50 and 70% of people with migraines have a family history of migraines (see figure 4).[4]

Robert's Story

Robert's story illustrates how the baffling variety of migraine symptoms can delay diagnosis and treatment. So can misconceptions.

Robert was 28 and had scarcely ever had a headache. His two sisters had both suffered from classic migraines

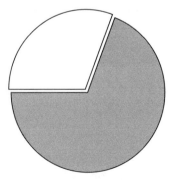

Figure 4. *Between 50 and 70% of all people with migraines have a family history of migraine headaches*

since their early teens. From discussions with them and with friends, Robert had mistakenly surmised that only women got migraines. He also assumed that all migraines were classic, like his sisters' were. Both of his sisters experienced auras, had pain located on only one side of the head, and experienced severe nausea during their migraine attacks.

When Robert first started experiencing headaches, they came without an aura or nausea, and he felt the pain all over his head. Naturally, he assumed that his headaches were caused by stress or perhaps a virus. In any event, Robert was certain of one thing. Although his headaches were extremely painful, they could not possibly be migraines: He wasn't a woman, and his headaches didn't resemble his sisters' classic migraines.

Robert's headaches continued to get worse, but the last thing he was about to do was visit his doctor and explain that he was suffering from a "woman's problem." It was only after he'd missed several days of work and endured a great deal of unnecessary pain that he finally sought his doctor's help for his headaches. It turned out that Robert was experiencing migraines—common migraines—and his doctor was able to prescribe medication that helped. Discovering the truth about migraines came as a great relief to Robert's aching skull and also to his shaken self-image.

How Do Doctors Diagnose Migraines?

As we've seen, migraine headaches can be difficult to diagnose. Classic migraines are the easiest to diagnose. An aura preceding a headache is the clearest sign of migraine. As we've seen, the intensity of the headache doesn't tell you whether or not the headache is a migraine. The type

Danger Signs

Headaches are painful, but they are usually not dangerous. However, rarely—in less than 3% of people with head-aches—a headache is a warning sign of a life-threatening problem such as a brain tumor, meningitis, an aneurysm, or a concussion. Such headaches are often characterized by excruciating pain that begins suddenly and persists, or recurs daily. Physical exertion will often intensify the pain.

The National Institute of Neurologic Disorders and Stroke recommends that you consult a physician immediately should you suffer from any of the following symptoms:

- A headache in combination with confusion, loss of consciousness, or convulsions

of pain may provide a helpful clue: Most (though not all) people who experience migraines describe the pain as pounding, pulsating, or throbbing, often in time with the heartbeat.

As we saw earlier, location is a fairly strong indication of a migraine. Sixty percent of migraines are located on just one side of the head, above or behind the eye. However, migraines can also occur virtually anywhere on the head, neck, and even shoulders, or they can spread to cover the entire head. It's also true that pain located on one side of the head, behind or above the eye, is not a foolproof sign of a migraine. Such pain can be caused by a sinus headache as well. (See chapter 9 for a discussion of sinus and other types of headache.)

Severe nausea and sensitivity to light, odors, and sound are two other strong indications of a migraine. Mild nausea can accompany many kinds of headaches as well

- A headache involving pain in the eye or ear

- A headache in combination with fever or nausea

- A headache occurring after a blow to the head

- A headache in combination with slurred speech, blurred vision, numbness, memory loss, or trouble walking

- A headache that grows worse, lasts longer than usual, or changes in nature

- A headache that is recurrent (especially in children)

- A headache that is persistent in someone who does not normally have headaches

migraines, but severe nausea is more typical of migraine headaches.

The more closely a migraine headache conforms to the classic pattern, the easier it is to diagnose. Doctors rely upon a few telltale signs for diagnosing a migraine.

1. Symptoms similar to an aura (as described above) preceding a headache.
2. Nausea and sensitivity to light, odors, and sound.
3. The location of pain on one half of the head (this is only important in combination with the other symptoms).
4. The nature of the pain itself. Though this method of diagnosis is the least definitive, in combination with the previous symptoms, it is often the sign of a migraine when the pain is pounding, pulsating, or throbbing in nature.

Finally, when doctors are puzzled by a hard-to-diagnose headache and have ruled out any serious health problems, they sometimes try prescribing a medication specific for migraines. If it works, then it's safe to conclude that the elusive headache was actually a migraine.

If you suspect you might have migraines but you've never been diagnosed, discuss the information in this chapter with your doctor or other health practitioner. You might also try feverfew or some of the other natural treatments discussed later in this book, on the same principle that doctors sometimes use: If the feverfew helps, then your headaches are probably migraines.

Warning: If you suffer from headaches, you should first consult with your doctor to rule out any potentially serious medical conditions. (See sidebar, Danger Signs.)

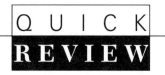

QUICK
REVIEW

- Migraine headaches are a specific kind of headache with a characteristic set of symptoms. The symptoms can be subtle, and the most characteristic symptoms are not always present.

- A typical migraine can last anywhere from several hours to several days.

- Migraine symptoms can vary from one person to the next, and migraine headaches are not always easy to diagnose.

- To diagnose a migraine headache, doctors need to carefully review the specific nature of your pain.

- When diagnosing your headache, your doctor will rely largely on your ability to describe the *intensity, duration, frequency, location,* and *type* of pain that you are experiencing.

- Besides headache pain, there are several other important symptoms of a migraine, including nausea and sensitivity to light, odors, and sound. Some people with migraines also experience diarrhea, fever, chills, or other symptoms.

- There are two types of migraine headache: *classic* and *common.* Classic migraines are preceded by an *aura,* which is a set of neurological symptoms such as visual disturbances, difficulty with speech, weakness in an arm or leg, tingling of the face or hands, dizziness, or general confusion. (Only about 20% of migraines fall into this category.) The rest are common migraines, whose symptoms can be more difficult to diagnose. Common migraines are not preceded by an aura.

- The intensity of most migraine headaches varies from moderate to severe.

- Some people experience migraines very rarely—perhaps only once every few years; others suffer a migraine as often as once or twice a week.

- Certain locations of pain are hallmarks of a migraine. Migraine headaches most often occur on one side of the head, just above or behind one eye. The side may change from migraine to migraine. In the course of a migraine attack, the pain can migrate from the original area of pain to another part of the head, neck, or shoulders.

- The most common type of pain described by people with migraines is a throbbing, pounding, or pulsating sensation. Following a migraine attack, people typically feel irritable and listless, with impaired concentration.

What Causes
a Migraine?

For many centuries, doctors have been struggling to understand what causes migraine headaches. Since the late nineteenth century, two major theories have been dominant. The *vascular theory* holds that migraine headaches are somehow caused by changes in blood vessels. The *neurological theory* holds that nerves are the primary cause of migraine headaches. Today, it is widely believed that both the nerves and the blood vessels that feed the brain are involved in the mechanism that causes migraine headaches, but there is much that we still don't understand.

The History of Nerve
and Blood Vessel Theories

The two major theories of migraine headaches have alternated in authority over the centuries (see figure 5).

In 1684, Dr. Thomas Willis attributed headaches to an increased blood flow to the brain. This blood flow,

Dr. Willis wrote, "distends the vessels, greatly blows up the membranes and pulls the nervous fibers one from another and so brings to them painful corrugations or wrinklings." This early version of the vascular theory explained many of the most striking features of a migraine. The throbbing quality of the pain seemed to indicate the throbbing of a distended blood vessel. Another feature of migraines that suggested a vascular cause was that the pain grew abruptly worse during mild physical activity, such as climbing a flight of stairs—an activity that would increase blood flow and thus add to the pressure on the distended vessel. Notice that while Dr. Willis did feel that nerves were involved, he thought that blood flow problems came first.

Today, it is widely believed that both the nerves and the blood vessels that feed the brain are involved in the mechanism that causes migraine headaches.

However, in the late nineteenth century, new theories focused on the nerves as the primary cause of migraines. In 1873, Dr. Liveing authored the first major modern work addressing migraines, *A Contribution to the Pathology of Nerve Storms*. In this influential treatise, Liveing argued that migraine headaches were very much like epileptic seizures. He believed that the vascular features of a migraine—the throbbing sensation and face discoloration—were actually secondary to "nerve storms."

In 1893, another physician, Dr. Gower, agreed. "We must not ascribe too much significance to throbbing, or to the increase in the pain by the causes of vascular distention," he said. "These may be due merely to the oversensitiveness of the central nervous structures."[1]

In the 1930s, the pendulum swung back when a pair of neurologists named John Graham and Harold Wolff redirected attention to the vascular features of migraines. The headache associated with migraines, they believed, was caused by the dilation of blood vessels outside the skull. They thought that the neurological symptoms of a migraine—namely the aura and related symptoms— were caused by the constriction of blood vessels inside the skull.

Neurological explanations then came to the fore again in the 1940s. A Harvard psychologist who himself suffered from migraines, Dr. Lashley, recorded his personal symptoms, and he described the aura as a castle passing across the field of vision. From his knowledge of the brain function, Lashley was able to estimate that an electrical change was proceeding across his *occipital cortex* (the part of the brain that controls vision) at a rate of 3 mm per minute.

Soon afterward, a Brazilian researcher, Dr. Leao, developed a theory about migraines based on his laboratory research involving electrical stimulation of the brains of rabbits. When he stimulated the visual region of the brain, he created a spreading pattern of electrical activity that reached the rabbits' *cerebral cortex,* an advanced part of the brain where migraine pain might be experienced. He theorized that a migraine headache might be a similar electrical event in the brain.

Four decades later, using more sophisticated tools, Dr. Welch was able to record such changes in electrical activity within the brains of people with migraines, as Dr. Leao's theory suggested.[2] Even more recent research has corroborated these findings.[3] The phenomenon of a spreading pattern of electrical activity in the brain (technically, a *spreading depression*) is believed by many today to be responsible for the slow march of castlelike images across the field of vision and other symptoms of the aura experienced by people with classic migraines.

In addition, Welch found that people with migraines had low levels of magnesium in certain parts of their brains at the beginning of an attack. Magnesium plays a role in nerve function, and magnesium deficiency may predispose individuals with migraines to abnormal electrical activity in the brain.[4] This may also explain why magnesium supplements seem to be helpful for migraines, as described in chapter 8.

However, the vascular explanation is far from dead. In the 1980s, Danish researchers discovered that many people with migraines experience a decrease in blood flow in the *occipital* region of the brain, the same area

Danish researchers discovered that many people with migraines experience a decrease in blood flow in the *occipital* region of the brain, the same area that controls vision.

that controls vision.[5] This decreased blood flow then slowly moves forward from this region and affects other areas of the cortex in the form of a wavelike, spreading decrease in blood flow (called *spreading oligemia*). The speed of this spreading change has been measured at 2 to 3 mm per minute—the same rate recorded by Dr. Lashley 40 years earlier! The decrease in blood flow can last for several hours.

Could it be that the change in blood flow is causing the spreading alteration in electrical activity? Or does the electrical activity change the blood flow? The nerves affect the blood vessels, the blood vessels affect the

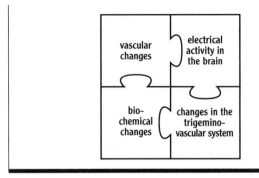

Figure 5. *The four major body changes associated with migraine headaches*

nerves, and both affect many other systems in the body. It's a chicken and egg situation.

To make matters even more complex, even the electrical theory of migraines has subtheories. While the research mentioned thus far has concentrated on the cerebral cortex, the more advanced portion of the brain, other evidence suggests that migraines may originate in some of the deeper, more primitive parts of the brain, the brainstem. A nerve in the face, the *trigeminal nerve,* may also play a role.

The nerves affect the blood vessels, the blood vessels affect the nerves, and both affect many other systems in the body.

Jill's Story

Jill is a 42-year-old accountant living in Boston. She began having migraines as an adolescent. Though some medications have helped, she still experiences a fairly severe attack at least once every couple of months.

She suffers from common rather than classic migraines. Her first sign of an impending headache is always a soft, rhythmic, slowly building pulsation near her temple. Before long, the pain grows to a throbbing crescendo. Jill can plainly sense that the throbbing pain follows the pattern of her pulse. Her children have told her that, when in the throes of an attack, she turns pale—her forehead can turn chalky white. Indeed, when they were younger, Jill's children found the sight of her writhing in pain truly frightening. They described her appearance as almost ghostly.

Jill's headaches illustrate why so many have held so strongly to a vascular explanation of migraines. The association of Jill's throbbing pain with the rhythm of her pulse seems patently obvious. Her pale appearance and chalky white forehead seem clearly linked to changes in her blood flow. Yet neither the vascular nor the nerve explanation can tell us the whole story of what Jill's symptoms mean. We must also consider the role of the brain chemical serotonin.

Beyond Nerves and Blood Vessels: The Neurotransmitters

In the last several decades, we have come to recognize the crucial role that certain chemicals such as serotonin play in the brain. It turns out that serotonin may also be linked to migraine attacks. Serotonin is a versatile neurotransmitter with a range of known and unknown functions. Among its known functions, serotonin is a potent *vasoconstrictor*—that is, it constricts blood vessels. This may well be one of its primary roles in a migraine attack. In addition to constricting blood vessels, serotonin is known to regulate pain messages and to help out with smooth muscle tissues and the digestive system. During a migraine, it is believed

A Menstrual Migraine

Debra is a 23-year-old graduate student who enjoys an active recreational life of camping, hiking, and rock-climbing. She began suffering migraine attacks after she turned 22. Her headaches follow a familiar pattern tied to her monthly menstrual period: Invariably, she suffers a vicious migraine attack on the first day of menstruation. Along with the pain of her throbbing head, Debra experiences occasional mood changes and sharp pain in her back. Before she began having migraines, Debra had never experienced mood changes or back pains during her menstrual period. Most perplexing of all for Debra is the fact that, other than during her menstrual period, she never experiences migraines or headaches of any sort.

that serotonin may work in combination with other bio-chemicals, such as neuropeptides, to sensitize blood vessel walls at the time of painful dilation.[6]

In order to relay messages between the brain and the nervous system, serotonin attaches to receptor sites, "docking" areas made to fit the molecule. There are four main families of serotonin receptors, each in its own part of the body. Two families of serotonin receptors are thought to be associated with migraine headaches: 5-HT1 and 5-HT2. Stimulating 5-HT1 receptors has been found to end a migraine attack that has begun. Blocking 5-HT2 receptors has been found to prevent a migraine. These findings may help explain how some antimigraine drugs work. As we will see in chapter 4, the migraine medication Imitrex stimulates 5-HT1 receptors. The migraine medications Sansert, Periactin, and some calcium channel–blockers block 5-HT2 receptors, among their many other

Debra's case is not unusual. Doctors have long known that there is an association between ovulation and migraine headaches, but we don't know exactly how this works. The most likely explanation is that a migraine can be triggered by fluctuations in the hormones *estrogen* and *progesterone*. Throughout a woman's menstrual cycle, her body's production of estrogen and progesterone rises and falls. One theory is that menstrual migraines are related to falling levels of estrogen.[7] Inflammatory substances called prostaglandins may also play a role.

actions.[8] There is some evidence that certain constituents of feverfew may affect serotonin as well, although the subject is far from clear. See chapter 5 for more information.

Other Biochemical Substances

Excitatory amino acids and other biochemical substances may also play a role in migraine headaches. Levels of *glutamate,* an excitatory amino acid, have shown to be elevated in people with migraines when they are between migraine episodes. This is especially true for people who experience auras.[9]

Prostaglandins may be partly responsible for the pain, inflammation, and dilation of blood vessels in menstrually related headaches. Prostaglandins are hormone-like molecules that control inflammatory processes in the body. *Nonsteroidal anti-inflammatory agents* such as Advil, Nuprin, Mediprin, and Motrin IB are known to be

What Triggers a Migraine?

S cience has identified many migraine "triggers." They fre-quently work in combination—in fact, a migraine is usually preceded by two or more of these factors. Potential migraine triggers include the following:

- food allergies
- food additives (nitrites, MSG, aspartame)
- dairy products
- chocolate
- nuts
- alcohol (especially red wine)
- caffeine (in excess, or caffeine withdrawal)
- stress or emotional changes
- disrupted sleep patterns

prostaglandin inhibitors. For this reason, as we will see in chapter 4, they can be an effective migraine treatment for people experiencing a menstrually related migraine. Menstrual migraines may also be related to levels of hormones such as *estrogen* and *progesterone* (see sidebar, A Menstrual Migraine).

Causes and Triggers

There is even one more factor to consider. Problems can have both deep causes and immediate triggers. Consider the Great Depression of the 1930s. While we don't under-stand everything that caused it, trade barriers and high taxes certainly played an immediate role in triggering the

- time zone changes
- exhaustion
- physical exertion
- missed meals
- loud noise
- bright or flickering lights
- perfumes
- poor posture
- muscle tension
- strong smells
- cigarette smoking
- weather changes
- eyestrain
- hormonal changes (menstruation, pregnancy, delivery)

crash. They alone probably didn't cause the worldwide economic collapse, but they certainly hastened it.

Similarly, migraines also have triggers, certain substances, actions, and stimuli that can set off the complex physiological reactions involved in a migraine headache. It is important to understand the difference between a trigger and a cause. A trigger alone cannot cause a migraine; a trigger is just one factor that somehow touches off a more complex interaction.

One thing is clear: Some people are predisposed to suffer migraines because of either their genes, their lifestyle and life experience, or some unknown combination of these factors. Triggers can only affect someone who has a predisposition to migraines.

So What *Really* Causes Migraines?

Nerves, blood vessels, brain chemicals, hormones, triggers: what does cause migraines? Modern-day experts can't agree on which one is most important. Actually, migraines may not have a single cause. To say that one thing "causes" something else implies a simple, direct relationship between the two things. It may not be possible to identify individual causes in a complex system like the brain. Was there a single "cause" of the Great Depression? Migraines may be at least as complex as international economic disasters. Fortunately, they seem to be easier to treat! See the upcoming chapters for options you can try, including the natural herb feverfew.

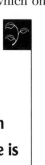

Modern-day experts can't agree on which migraine cause is most important. Actually, migraines may not have a single cause.

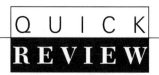

QUICK
REVIEW

- Our understanding of migraine headaches today may be described as sophisticated yet incomplete.
- Current research emphasizes three basic types of physical changes associated with a migraine headache: vascular changes; electrical activity in the brain, brainstem, and trigeminal nerve; and biochemical changes.

- During a migraine, waves of changing blood flow and nerve activity travel through the brain.
- The brain chemical serotonin appears to play a major role in migraine headaches.
- A number of factors, such as alcohol or lack of sleep, can trigger a migraine.
- All these factors probably interact to produce the problem we call a migraine headache.

Conventional Treatment for Migraine Headaches

Conventional treatment for migraines today isn't perfect, but it offers many useful and effective options. The drug sumatriptan (Imitrex), for example, appears to relieve a migraine attack for about 85% of people who take it, and other treatments can be taken on a daily basis for prevention. This chapter will describe how today's conventional treatments came to be developed and will discuss in detail their strengths and weaknesses. (If you wish to skip ahead to read about natural treatments for migraines, please see chapters 5, 6, 7, and 8.)

Historical Treatments for Migraines

Reports of migraines go back thousands of years. The ancient Greeks first coined the term *hemikrania,* meaning "half of the head," to reflect migraine's peculiar tendency to afflict just one half of the skull. The French word *migraine,* which we use today, had its origins in the Greek term.

Migraines are cruelly painful. Up until about 100 years ago, however, the treatments were often worse than the headaches, and are almost unbelievable today. Perhaps the mildest was blood-letting, a popular treatment for migraines through the nineteenth century. Blood-letting, at one time a standard treatment for many ailments, was thought to cleanse and purify the body and thus relieve a variety of conditions. For those whose headache did not respond well to this initial treatment, the treatment of choice was often a second blood-letting.

If blood-letting didn't work, the real suffering at the hands of doctors began. A medieval person with a migraine might be referred to a specialist who would apply a hot iron to the site of the

The ancient Greeks coined the term *hemikrania*, meaning "half of the head," to reflect migraine's peculiar tendency to afflict just one half of the skull.

pain. While this treatment may or may not have been effective—no modern researchers have studied it experimentally(!)—the side effects were thought rather extreme even by medieval standards. They included permanent facial scarring, severe trauma, and temporary blindness. (However, we can assume that there was very little risk of addiction.)

If the hot iron to the head did not do the trick, a medieval person with a migraine might have submitted to another extreme treatment: having a hole drilled in the skull to free the evil spirits that were presumed to cause the headache. Side effects included excessive bleeding, permanent brain damage, and not infrequently, death.

Migraine Medications

Migraine Relief

- sumatriptan (Imitrex)
- ergotamine (Bellergal-S, Cafergot, Wigraine)
- dihydroergotamine (DHE-45)
- nonprescription nonsteroidal anti-inflammatories: ibuprofen (Advil, Nuprin, Mediprin, Motrin IB)
- prescription nonsteroidal anti-inflammatories: naproxen sodium (Anaprox), flurbiprofen (Ansaid), ketoprofen (Orudis), meclofenamate (Meclomen), ketorolac (Toradol), diclofenac sodium (Volaren), indomethacin (Indocin)
- over-the-counter analgesics: acetylsalicylic acid (aspirin), acetaminophen (Tylenol), acetylsalicylic acid/acetaminophen (Excedrin)
- combination analgesics: acetaminophen dichloralphenazone isometheptene (Midrin), aspirin/caffeine/butalbital (Fiorinal)
- opiates: codeine, butorphanol (Stadol), meperidine (Demerol)

Finally, if none of these treatments worked, our battered individual could turn to yet another desperate treatment: having a clove of garlic inserted into the temple, through an incision. Side effects from this "treatment" included excessive bleeding, infection, trauma, and an occasional death.

Anyone who's had a severe migraine can understand why people suffering from migraines would re-

- antiemetics: ondansetron (Zofran), metoclopramide (Reglan), promethazine (Phenergan), prochlorperazine (Compazine), trimethobenzamide (Tigan)

Migraine Prevention

- beta-blockers: propranolol hydrochloride (Inderal, Inderal-LA), nadolol (Corgard), timolol (Blocadren), atenolol (Tenormin), metoprolol (Lopressor)
- preventive ergot drugs: methysergide maleate (Sansert), methylergonovine (Methergine)
- calcium channel blockers: verapamil (Calan, Isoptin, Verelan, Covera-HS), diltiazem (Cardizem), isradipine (DynaCirc), nicardipine (Cardene), nimodipine (Nimotop), nifedipine (Procardia, Adalt), propranol hydrochloride (Inderal)
- antidepressants
- selective serotonin-reuptake inhibitors (SSRIs): fluoxetine (Prozac), sertraline (Zoloft), paroxetine (Paxil)
- monoamine oxidase inhibitors: phenelzine (Nardil), isocarboxazid (Marplan)

sort to such extreme treatments. However, not all folk treatments were so punishing. Although its use isn't well documented, we know that the herb feverfew survived as a gentle folk remedy for migraines in England for centuries.

The modern drug treatment of migraine headaches began in the late nineteenth century with the ergot drugs, agents that are still used today.

Modern Drug Treatments for Migraines

The past few decades have seen great advances in the treatment of migraine headaches, and new pharmaceuticals have brought substantial relief to people with migraines. To fully understand the many options available for the treatment of migraine headaches, we need to look at four areas:

1. The different kinds of drugs.
2. How each of the drugs works.
3. How effective the drugs are at preventing or alleviating migraines.
4. What, if any, side effects you may experience when taking them.

There are two basic types of migraine medications. Some provide *relief* during a migraine, while others *prevent* future migraines. The herb feverfew falls in the latter category.

Migraine relief medications need to be taken at the first sign of an approaching headache to help alleviate the pain of an attack.

Migraine Relief Medications

Migraine relief medications help alleviate the pain of an attack once it's started. These medications need to be taken at the first sign of an approaching headache. There are two kinds of conventional migraine relief medication: drugs that are specifically designed for migraines, and drugs that have more general uses as pain relievers (see sidebar, Migraine Medications, for a complete listing of relief medications).

Migraine-specific medications all target serotonin. As we saw in chapter 3, serotonin is a neurotransmitter that plays a role in migraine headaches. Many migraine relief medications stimulate the 5-HT1 family of serotonin receptors in the nerves, blood vessels, and brainstem that receive serotonin molecules. These drugs include *sumatriptan* (Imitrex), *ergotamine* (Bellergal-S, Cafergot, Wigraine), and *dihydroergotamine* (DHE 45). (The ergot drugs actually have many other effects as well that may be equally or more important; sumatriptan is very specific.)

The general pain relievers used for migraine include analgesics such as aspirin and Tylenol; nonsteroidal anti-inflammatory medications such as ibuprofen; combination analgesics such as Midrin and Fiorinal; and, in severe cases, an injection of Demerol or another opiate. For a comparison of benefits and side effects of migraine relief medications, see table 1 on page 56.

> **Since its introduction in 1993, sumatriptan has been hailed as a revolutionary advance in migraine relief medication.**

Sumatriptan

Since its introduction in 1993, sumatriptan has been hailed as a revolutionary advance in migraine relief medication. Most migraine medications seem to work consistently for about half the individuals who try them, or fewer. Sumatriptan, in contrast, helps 70 to 85% of people.[1,2] Of all the pharmaceuticals available today, sumatriptan comes closest to being universally effective.

Like the ergot drugs ergotamine and dihydroergotamine, sumatriptan stimulates the 5-HT1 family of

Know Your Rights

Before you consider conventional migraine treatments, it is important that you know what you have a right to expect. The American Council on Headache Education has endorsed the following Migraineur's Bill of Rights.[3]

1. I have the right to be taken seriously by my physician when I go for treatment of my headaches.
2. I have the right to a complete and thorough medical examination, including a medical history and complete neurological evaluation.
3. I have the right to appropriate diagnostic testing, including neurodiagnostics, CT scans, and MRI scans, if necessary, when my headaches are first evaluated and when the headache pattern or severity changes.
4. I have the right to be referred to a specialist—for example, a neurologist, a headache specialist, or a headache clinic—if my headaches do not respond to my primary physician's treatment, or if my primary physician feels a specialist's care is needed.

serotonin receptors—in particular, a subset known as the 5-HT1D receptors. This causes the blood vessels to constrict, thus reducing inflammation and pressure on the nerves. But sumatriptan is a modern "designer drug" that acts much more selectively than either of these earlier medications.[4] Ergot drugs affect numerous parts of the body, while sumatriptan targets one very specific receptor on blood vessels. As a consequence, it has fewer side effects.

5. I have the right to receive specific headache therapy, if needed, instead of nonprescription drugs, narcotics, or combination analgesics that may increase the problem.

6. I have the right to return for additional help whenever my treatment plan seems to be inadequate to control my headaches.

7. I have the right to be treated courteously and responsibly in emergency rooms, if a severe headache fails to respond to my usual treatment plan.

8. I have the right to expect my insurance company to recognize migraine as a legitimate illness, and to persist in appealing any denied claims for legitimate medical care that would be covered for other illnesses.

9. I have the right to expect those around me—family, friends, coworkers, and others who come in contact with me—to make an effort to understand my illness and to cooperate with me in my efforts to live a full, rich life.

Sumatriptan also acts rapidly. One study found injected sumatriptan relieved pain within about 41 minutes.[5] (The oral form of this drug takes longer to relieve migraines.) However, it's important to note that even sumatriptan doesn't necessarily wipe out all vestiges of pain from a migraine. For many people, effective relief may mean only that their headache is significantly less intense than it would have been without the medication, but not gone altogether. The degree of relief varies; some individuals might have their pain reduced by 80% or more, while others might experience only about a 50% reduction in pain. Furthermore, for some people, migraines have a nasty habit of coming back within 24 hours after a pain-relief medication has been used. In this case, a second dose of sumatriptan is generally effective.

Sumatriptan is only effective if it's taken after the headache pain has begun. When taken during the aura phase, for example, sumatriptan will not have any impact on the head pain that follows. If used correctly, however, sumatriptan is an effective treatment for many people. It not only relieves headache pain; it also seems to reduce post-headache lassitude and the frequency of headaches somewhat. Also, evidence suggests that it does not lose its effectiveness when used frequently.

> **If used correctly, sumatriptan is an effective treatment for many people. It not only relieves headache pain; it also seems to reduce post-headache lassitude and the frequency of headaches somewhat.**

Originally, sumatriptan had to be taken as an injection—which meant that people with migraines who used it had to learn to inject themselves. Now it is also available in oral form, which is much easier for most people to take, and in a nasal spray that takes effect more quickly than the oral form.

Although most people can safely take it, sumatriptan can cause side effects. These may include increased heart rate; elevated blood pressure; and tightness in the chest, jaw, or neck.

Warning: Because sumatriptan constricts blood vessels, people with heart disease (or at high risk for it) should only take sumatriptan under the close supervision of a doctor. In general, you are at high risk for heart disease if you smoke, if you have a family history of coronary artery disease, if your cholesterol level is high, or if you suffer from hypertension or obesity. (For information on treatments for heart disease, see *The Natural Pharmacist Guide to Heart Disease Prevention*.)

Ergotamine and Dihydroergotamine

In the past five years, drugs derived in the ergot family have been eclipsed by sumatriptan. But ergotamine and dihydroergotamine are still effective treatments for many people.

Interestingly, a new form of the dihydroergotamine earned positive notoriety during the 1998 Super Bowl when the Denver Broncos' running back, Terrell Davis, suffered a migraine during the game. The rapid action of the nasal spray form of this old but effective drug sparked his second-half efforts that led to the Broncos' victory.

Ergotamine must be taken at the very onset of migraine pain to work. It can be taken orally, by injection, as a nasal spray, or as a suppository.

Ergotamine drugs act on a wide variety of receptor sites in the brain, producing numerous, contradictory, and poorly understood effects. The result of this potpourri of influences is constriction of blood vessels and prevention of a full-blown migraine attack. Ergotamine must be taken at the very onset of migraine pain to work. It can be taken orally, by injection, as a nasal spray, or as a suppository.

Ergotamine is effective for nearly half of those who try it, but it has a troublesome side effect: The majority of people who take it become nauseated.[6] Since migraines themselves cause nausea, this is an extremely unpleasant side effect.

Besides nausea, ergotamine's other possible side effects include vomiting, stomach or muscle cramps, tingling and swelling in the arms or legs, and "rebound headaches." The latter are not migraines but simply a type of headache that is caused by taking a lot of headache medication and then stopping. As with Imitrex, people with severe atherosclerosis, coronary artery disease, and high blood pressure should not use ergotamine, because it constricts arteries.

> **With dihydroergotamine there's more leeway than with ergotamine: you don't have to catch the migraine right at the beginning.**

Dihydroergotamine is a modified form of ergotamine. Like ergotamine, dihydroergotamine stimulates 5-HT1 serotonin receptors, as well as producing many other changes in the brain.[7] With dihydroergotamine there's more leeway than with ergotamine: you don't have to catch the migraine right at the beginning. Another advantage is that it is less apt to cause nausea and rebound headaches. Dihydroergotamine can be taken either orally or by injection.

There are a few specific side effects associated with the use of dihydroergotamine. The most common are nasal stuffiness and muscle cramps (particularly stomach

Lisa's Story

Lisa was a hospital nurse. Since her late twenties, Lisa had suffered from migraine headaches. For nearly a decade, she had been using Bellergal-S, a standard ergotamine medication, to relieve her migraine pain. She was also using Phenergan, an antiemetic, to control her nausea. Unfortunately, Bellergal-S was only somewhat helpful. It reduced the intensity of her migraines, but not enough.

Even with the Bellergal-S, Lisa's headaches were intense enough to force her to leave work and rest in a quiet, dark room. After her migraine had passed, Lisa felt an overwhelming sense of weakness and fatigue. Bellergal-S allowed Lisa to function, but she remained very much at the mercy of her migraines.

In late 1994, Lisa read an article about the "miraculous" new migraine drug, sumatriptan. In March 1995, largely because of Lisa's prompting, her doctor switched her from Bellergal-S to Imitrex (the brand name for sumatriptan). The impact on Lisa's headaches was immediate and decisive. At the first sign of pain, Lisa injected herself with Imitrex; in less than 30 minutes, her pain was entirely relieved. The sumatriptan also relieved her nausea and post-headache malaise.

cramps), symptoms that are less likely to occur when using ergotamine or sumatriptan. Again, people with coronary disease (or at high risk for it) should only use dihydroergotamine under the supervision of a physician.

Nonsteroidal Anti-Inflammatories (NSAIDs)

Nonsteroidal anti-inflammatory drugs (NSAIDs) can alleviate the symptoms of acute migraine attacks. Some NSAIDs, such as aspirin and ibuprofen, can be purchased over the counter at any drugstore. For others, such as indomethacin, you need a prescription. There are many other NSAIDs available, but they all work essentially the same way: by inhibiting the body's production of inflammatory compounds called prostaglandins.[8] Prostaglandins play a major role in both inflammation and pain.

The effectiveness of different NSAIDs tends to vary greatly among individual people with migraines.[9] There is no single standout drug; what works for one person may not work as well for another, and vice versa. You may want to try up to three different NSAIDs before you draw any conclusions about whether this class of medication can help you.[10] In general, NSAIDs are useful for mild to moderate migraine pain and may be particularly effective for menstrual cycle–related migraines.

In general, NSAIDs are useful for mild to moderate migraine pain and may be particularly effective for menstrual cycle–related migraines.

The major problem with NSAIDs is that they irritate the stomach, potentially causing bleeding or even perforated ulcers. However, severe stomach problems usually don't develop except after long-term, continual use. Occasional use for migraines shouldn't cause this problem. Other potential side effects include indigestion, lightheadedness, dizziness, diarrhea, and kidney or liver damage. Additionally, some studies have found that a significant number of people who take NSAIDs experience rebound headaches.[11]

Warning: People with ulcer disease, asthma, or clotting disorders should use NSAIDs only under a doctor's close supervision, if at all.

Over-the-Counter Analgesics

Along with the nonprescription NSAIDs, over-the-counter pain medications such as acetaminophen (Tylenol) and combination therapies such as Excedrin (aspirin, acetaminophen, and caffeine) are the first remedies that most people with migraines try. For many people, especially those who have mild migraines, these analgesics can be quite effective.[12,13]

However, over-the-counter analgesics can have potentially dangerous side effects. It may seem that a medication you can buy at any grocery store would be too mild to cause harm, but in fact these medications are not always the best choice for long-term use. For example, while acetaminophen has virtually no immediate side effects, if it's used in excess over time—especially in combination with alcohol—it can injure the liver. Excedrin contains aspirin, which like any other NSAID can damage the stomach.

In general, if you find yourself relying regularly on an over-the-counter medication, you should consult your doctor to see if there's a better long-term treatment for you.

Combination Analgesics
Available by Prescription

The drug Midrin combines acetaminophen with *dichloralphenazone* and *isometheptene*. Dichloralphenazone is a mild tranquilizer; isometheptene is a special amine, or nitrogen-containing compound, that constricts blood vessels. Studies have indicated that Midrin can be an effective migraine headache treatment.[14,15] Specific side effects associated with the use of Midrin include drowsiness, dizziness, skin rash, and gastrointestinal symptoms.

Fiorinal is another combination analgesic, containing aspirin, caffeine, and butalbital. Butalbital is a short-acting barbiturate that has been found to be very effective for migraines when taken early in an attack.[16] Caffeine combined with analgesics has been found to significantly enhance their effectiveness. However, all barbiturate-containing drugs have potential drawbacks, including rebound headaches and addiction.

The possible side effects of Fiorinal include drowsiness, hyperactivity, memory loss, and confusion. You should not drive or do anything that requires alertness when taking Fiorinal. Also, you should never combine Fiorinal with alcohol.

> **Opiates are a powerful class of painkillers that can provide immediate relief from severe and debilitating migraine attacks.**

Opiates

Opiates are a powerful class of painkillers that can provide immediate relief from severe and debilitating migraine attacks. Unfortunately, they are highly addictive and are generally prescribed only on an occasional basis for excruciating pain.[17]

Although opiates are not a good long-term treatment for migraine headaches, they may bring rapid relief for someone suffering a debilitating migraine attack. Opiates can be taken orally, by injection, or via nasal spray.

Some examples of opiates include codeine, butorphanol (Stadol), and meperidine (Demerol). Aside from addiction, the side effects associated with opiates include nausea, drowsiness, dizziness, constipation, and rebound headaches.

Antiemetics (Antinausea Medications)

Antiemetics are not designed to provide direct relief for the migraine itself. Rather, this class of medications relieves the nausea that often accompanies migraine headaches. Antiemetics were not originally designed with treating migraine headaches in mind, but they have been tremendously useful to those who experience migraines. Another advantage of antiemetics is that they can help people with migraines handle oral headache medication without feeling sick.[18,19] Some examples of antiemetics include ondansetron (Zofran), metoclopramide (Reglan), promethazine (Phenergan), prochlorperazine (Compazine), and trimethobenzamide (Tigan).

Antiemetics can be taken orally, as a suppository, or in the form of an injection, and they are extremely effective in relieving nausea for almost everyone who takes them. For some individuals experiencing migraines, this kind of medication relieves nausea entirely; for others, the

Antiemetics can be taken orally, as a suppository, or in the form of an injection, and they are extremely effective in relieving nausea.

nausea is reduced but not completely eliminated. Antiemetics may be especially useful for those who rely on

Table 1. Comparison of
Migraine Relief Medications

Migraine Relief Medication	Possible Benefits	Possible Side Effects
Sumatriptan (Imitrex)	helps 70 to 85% of those who take it closest to being universally effective acts rapidly may reduce post-headache lassitude and headache frequency maintains effectiveness when used frequently	increased heart rate elevated blood pressure tightness in chest, jaw, or neck
Ergotamine (Bellergal-S, Cafergot, Wigraine)	effective for nearly 50% of those who take it	nausea/vomiting stomach or muscle cramps tingling and swelling in arms or legs rebound headaches
Dihydroergotamine (DHE-45)	acts rapidly less apt to cause nausea than ergotamine; more leeway than with ergotamine (don't have to catch the headache right at the beginning)	nasal stuffiness muscle cramps (particularly stomach cramps)

Table 1. Comparison of Migraine Relief Medications *(continued)*

Migraine Relief Medication	Possible Benefits	Possible Side Effects
Nonsteroidal Anti-Inflammatories (aspirin, ibuprofen, indomethacin, Advil, Nuprin, Mediprin, Motrin IB)	can alleviate symptoms of acute migraine attacks useful for mild to moderate migraine pain particularly effective for menstrual cycle–related migraines	stomach irritation (potentially causes bleeding or even perforated ulcers) indigestion lightheadedness dizziness diarrhea kidney or liver damage rebound headaches
Over-the-Counter Analgesics (Tylenol, Excedrin)	effective for most migraines	potential liver injury (if used in excess over time) potential stomach damage
Combination Analgesics Available by Prescription (Midrin, Fiorinal)	effective for most migraines	drowsiness dizziness skin rash gastrointestinal symptoms potential rebound headaches potential addiction hyperactivity memory loss confusion

(continues)

Table 1. Comparison of Migraine Relief Medications *(continued)*

Migraine Relief Medication	Possible Benefits	Possible Side Effects
Opiates (codeine, Stadol, Demerol)	can provide immediate relief from debilitating migraines	highly addictive not good for long-term treatment nausea drowsiness dizziness constipation rebound headaches
Antiemetics (antinausea medications such as Zofran, Reglan, Phenergan, Compazine, Tigan)	relieves nausea that often accompanies migraines helps people with migraines handle oral headache medication without feeling sick	drowsiness dry mouth dizziness abnormal involuntary movements reduced blood pressure

Table 2. Comparison of
Migraine Prevention Medications

Migraine Prevention Medication	Possible Benefits	Possible Side Effects
Beta-Blockers (Inderal, Inderal-LA, Corgard, Blocadren, Tenormin, Lopressor)	reduce intensity and frequency of most migraines decrease duration of migraines successful for 60% of those who take them	lower blood pressure slow heartbeat cause airways to constrict may be unsuitable for diabetics because they interfere with key warning signals of an insulin reaction (sweating, anxiety, and increased heart rate) fatigue depression impotence worsened asthma reduced blood pressure lowered pulse rate dizziness weight gain gastrointestinal symptoms cold hands and feet nightmares

(continues)

Table 2. Comparison of Migraine Prevention Medications *(continued)*

Migraine Relief Medication	Possible Benefits	Possible Side Effects
Ergot Drugs (Sansert, Methergine)	successful for 60% of those who take them	nausea muscle cramps abdominal pain blood circulation problems weight gain leg cramps
Calcium Channel Blockers (Calan, Isoptin, Verelan, Covera-HS, Cardizem, DynaCirc, Cardene, Nimotop, Procardia, Adalt, cardene)	reduce intensity and decrease duration of most migraines	constipation fluid retention drowsiness cardiac dysfunction headaches

ergotamine drugs for migraine prevention since anti-emetics can cause nausea themselves.

The specific side effects associated with antiemetics include drowsiness, dry mouth, dizziness, abnormal involuntary movements, and reduced blood pressure. A new drug called ondansetron (Zofran) works in a very different way and offers potential advantages in terms of effectiveness and side effects. Unfortunately, at present it is very expensive.

Table 2. Comparison of Migraine
Prevention Medications

Migraine Relief Medication	Possible Benefits	Possible Side Effects
Antidepressants (selective serotonin-reuptake inhibitors/ SSRIs such as Prozac, Zoloft, Paxil)	prevent severe and persistent migraine headaches	nausea insomnia sexual disturbances fatigue mild agitation or nervousness headaches
Antidepressants (monoamine oxidase inhibitors/ MAOIs, such as Nardil, Marplan)	prevent severe and persistent migraine headaches possibly successful for 80% of those who take them	can be potentially fatal when combined with many other medications as well as certain foods insomnia weight gain severe changes in blood pressure

Migraine Prevention Medications

The medications discussed in the previous section of this chapter are all designed to provide relief from a migraine after an attack has begun. This is all well and good for those who suffer only occasional migraines. But people who have frequent migraines would be better off finding a medication to prevent the migraines from happening in the first place. The rest of this chapter will describe the

Migraine Prevention and Diet

In chapter 3 we saw that certain foods are migraine triggers for many people. Many people find significant relief without drugs, simply through avoiding trigger foods in their diets. It may take trial and error to determine which of these substances, if any, act as triggers for you.

Foods containing any of the following chemicals have been identified as potential migraine triggers:

- tyramine (found in yogurt, figs, bananas, freshly baked bread, red wine, cheeses, and fava beans)
- phenylethylamines (found in chocolate and decongestants such as Sudafed)
- nitrates (hot dogs, bologna, salami, bacon)
- monosodium glutamate (potato chips, canned meats/soups, prepared diet foods, prepared food from some Chinese restaurants, salad dressings)
- aspartame (NutraSweet)
- alcohol (especially red wine and beer)
- avocados and peanuts

available medicines that aim to do just that, sometimes known as migraine prophylactics. (As we will see in chapters 5 and 8, the herb feverfew and the supplement magnesium also seem to help prevent migraines.)

Migraine prophylactics come in four basic categories:

1. *Beta-blockers* are the most widely prescribed preventive medication for migraines, and they have proven to be highly effective at reducing the frequency of migraine headaches.

2. *Ergot drugs* are among the oldest migraine prevention medications and can also be very effective.

3. *Calcium channel–blockers* are less popular than either beta-blockers or ergot drugs due to certain side effects, but they too have been shown to reduce the incidence of migraines.

4. *Antidepressants*—in particular, *selective serotonin—reuptake inhibitors* and *monoamine oxidase inhibitors*—appear to be effective in some people but have not been thoroughly studied.

As with many migraine relief medications, migraine prevention medications work with varying success for different people. For this reason, your doctor may suggest that you try more than one to discover which is the most effective for you. It has been estimated that there is, at best, a 60 to 75% probability of success with any one medication designed to prevent migraines.[20] Success is defined as a significant reduction in the frequency of occurrence and the intensity of pain. In other words, prophylactic medications usually can't completely eliminate all migraine headaches, but they can

It has been estimated that there is, at best, a 60 to 75% probability of success with any one medication. Success is defined as a significant reduction in the frequency of occurrence and the intensity of pain.

significantly reduce the intensity and frequency of headaches. Such medications can reduce a debilitating medical condition to a nuisance. For a comparison of benefits and side effects of migraine relief medications, see table 2.

Beta-Blockers

Beta-blockers are among the most commonly prescribed migraine prevention medications. Though beta-blockers cannot stop all migraines from occurring, they are prescribed to reduce migraines' intensity and frequency and decrease their duration.

> **Prophylactic medications usually can't completely eliminate all migraine headaches, but they can significantly reduce the intensity and frequency of headaches.**

As with many drugs, their use as preventive medication for migraines was based on an accidental discovery. In the late 1960s a person was taking beta-blockers to treat his heart disease. After extended use, he noticed that his migraines had inexplicably disappeared. This discovery led to a battery of clinical trials to test the effectiveness of beta-blockers as an antimigraine medication.

Today, the effectiveness of beta-blockers in preventing migraines has been well established. There is generally a 60% success rate (a significant reduction in the frequency and/or intensity of a person's migraines).[21] Beta-blockers are thought to be able to prevent migraine headaches by stabilizing serotonin levels and stopping certain receptor nerves from dilating blood vessels.

Some caution is warranted in the use of beta-blockers because they have a wide range of effects on the heart, blood vessels, lungs, and central nervous system. Beta-blockers lower blood pressure. They can also slow the heartbeat and cause the airways to constrict. For these reasons people with heart disease may not be able to use beta-blockers. Another effect of these medications may make them unsuitable for diabetics: They interfere with some of the body's key warning signals of an insulin reaction, such as sweating, anxiety, and increased heart rate.

Some caution is warranted in the use of beta-blockers because they have a wide range of effects on the heart, blood vessels, lungs, and central nervous system. For these reasons, people with heart disease may not be able to use beta-blockers.

Some of the beta-blockers used for migraines are propranolol hydrochloride (Inderal, Inderal-LA), nadolol (Corgard), timolol (Blocadren), atenolol (Tenormin), and metoprolol (Lopressor). Specific side effects associated with the use of beta-blockers include fatigue, depression, impotence, worsened asthma, reduced blood pressure and a lowered pulse rate, dizziness, weight gain, gastrointestinal symptoms, cold hands and feet, and nightmares.

Ergot Drugs for Prevention

Certain ergot derivatives are used for the prevention of migraine headaches rather than treatment. Studies have found that ergotamine drugs are effective in 60% of those who take them.[22] The main ergotamine drugs used for prevention are methysergide maleate (Sansert) and methylergonovine (Methergine). Side effects associated with the use of these drugs include nausea, muscle cramps, pain, blood circulation problems, weight gain, and leg cramps.

Calcium Channel–Blockers

Like beta-blockers and ergot drugs, calcium channel–blockers are migraine prevention medications that have

> **Calcium channel blockers are migraine prevention medications that have also been shown to reduce the intensity and decrease the duration of migraines.**

also been shown to reduce the intensity and decrease the duration of migraines. The precise mechanism by which calcium channel–blockers prevent migraines is not certain.[23] One theory is that these medications reduce the frequency of migraines by decreasing arterial spasms.[24]

Calcium channel–blockers are generally not as effective as beta-blockers in preventing migraines, and effectiveness varies between specific drugs.[25] However, they may have fewer side effects for certain people.

The calcium channel–blockers include verapamil (Calan, Isoptin, Verelan, Covera-HS), diltiazem (Cardizem), isradipine (DynaCirc), nicardipine (Cardene), nimodipine (Nimotop), nifedipine (Procardia, Adalt), and cardene. Specific side effects associated with the use of these medications include constipation, fluid retention, drowsiness, cardiac dysfunction, and in some cases, headaches.

Warning: People with certain heart conditions may not be able to use calcium channel–blockers. If you have a heart condition, your doctor can advise you in choosing a migraine prevention medication.

Michelle's Story

Michelle had suffered from moderate to severe migraine headaches since she was a teenager. Unfortunately, the migraine medications her doctor prescribed for her gave her only minimal relief. After 5 years of limited results from using ergotamine, Michelle's doctor switched her to dihydroergotamine. While this medication was slightly more effective, Michelle still suffered a great deal of headache pain.

Her doctor wanted to prescribe beta-blockers to prevent Michelle's migraines, but Michelle had severe asthma. After one bad reaction to the beta-blockers had landed her in the emergency room, she was advised not to try the medication again. Michelle briefly tried ergot drugs but again met with little success.

Her doctor had never seen particularly strong results for her patients with migraines who tried calcium channel–blockers. But little else seemed to be helping Michelle, so the doctor prescribed a calcium channel–blocker (Calan) for her on a trial basis. On this medication, Michelle finally began to experience genuine relief. Aside from some swelling of the hands and feet, Michelle found it very effective and nearly free of side effects. Both the frequency and the severity of Michelle's migraine attacks subsided. Michelle, like many people with migraines, had to endure a lengthy process of trial and error before she found a medication that worked for her without causing serious side effects.

Antidepressants

Antidepressants are prescribed to prevent severe and persistent migraine headaches. It's not that migraine headaches are caused by depression. Rather, certain antidepressants affect serotonin levels and may thereby help prevent migraines as a kind of positive side effect.

MAOI drugs are also effective, but they are rather dangerous. They can interact seriously, even potentially fatally, with a great many other medications as well as certain foods. For this reason, they are not commonly prescribed for migraine prevention except as a last resort.

Remember, serotonin plays a significant role in migraine headaches.[26,27] The two major types of antidepressants that appear to be helpful for migraine prevention are *selective serotonin-reuptake inhibitors (SSRIs)* and *monoamine oxidase inhibitors (MAOIs)*.

SSRIs include fluoxetine (Prozac), sertraline (Zoloft), and paroxetine (Paxil). Dosage levels for effective migraine prevention are often below those required for depression. Side effects associated with SSRIs include nausea, insomnia, sexual disturbances, fatigue, mild agitation or nervousness, and headaches. When used for migraine prevention, very low doses may be sufficient, and at such doses side effects may be less common.

The MAOI drugs are also effective, but they are rather dangerous. They can interact seriously, even potentially fatally, with a great many other medications as well as certain foods. For this reason, they are not commonly prescribed for migraine prevention except as a last resort. However, it has been reported that 80% of people with migraines who take MAOIs experience significant improvement.[28]

MAOIs sometimes prescribed to prevent migraines include phenelzine (Nardil) and isocarboxazid (Marplan). The side effects of MAOIs are significantly more serious than those for the SSRIs. These side effects include insomnia, weight gain, and severe changes in blood pressure. It is critical that you closely follow your physician's instructions with respect to which foods and medications to avoid when using MAOIs.

Q U I C K
R E V I E W

- Migraine medications can be divided into two categories. Migraine *relief* medications are designed to put an end to an attack once it's begun. Migraine *prevention* medications are designed to stop an attack from occurring.

- There is a growing number of migraine relief medications, some of which have been developed specifically to treat migraines and others that have applications beyond migraines.

- *Sumatriptan, ergotamine,* and *dihydroergotamine* can all relieve migraine symptoms. Nonsteroidal anti-inflammatories (NSAIDs), over-the-counter analgesics, combination analgesics, opiates, and antiemetics may be helpful as well.

- Opiates are powerful painkillers that are prescribed to provide immediate relief from occasional, severe migraine attacks.

- Migraine prevention medications generally fall into four categories: *beta-blockers, ergot drugs, calcium channel–blockers,* and *antidepressants.*
- Antidepressant drugs may also help prevent migraines.

CHAPTER
FIVE

Feverfew
The Scientific Evidence

I n this chapter, we will need to carefully separate what we *know* from what we merely *suspect*. This means understanding the difference between scientific evidence and anecdotal reports.

Many people with migraines have taken feverfew and reported that their migraines grew less frequent and intense or stopped altogether.

We know that many people with migraines have taken feverfew and reported that their migraines grew less frequent and intense or stopped altogether. We therefore suspect that some component of the feverfew plant can prevent and relieve migraine headaches. But such anecdotal reports—that is, individual stories as opposed to the results of methodical research—can be misleading. You really need scientific studies to know whether a treatment works. As we will see in this chapter, the research evidence for feverfew (at least when taken in leaf form) is generally positive, but more studies are needed.

This chapter walks you through the steps of medical research and shows how far the study of feverfew's effectiveness for migraines has progressed.

What Makes a Study Valid?

Whether it's a drug or an herb, a new treatment needs to be validated scientifically. Before a treatment is accepted, three questions need to be answered:

1. Is the treatment effective?
2. What is the appropriate dosage, and in what form should it be taken?
3. Is the treatment safe?

> **Whether it's a drug or an herb, a new treatment needs to be validated scientifically.**

Over the past several decades, conventional medicine has developed standard procedures for evaluating whether a treatment is effective. Natural treatments should be held to an equally high standard. The way to answer these questions is to use the scientific method: to form hypotheses and test them in rigorously designed studies.

The Qualities of a Well-Designed Study

In order to have valid results, a scientific experiment must have four qualities. It must be repeatable, placebo controlled double-blind, and randomized.

When we say that an experiment is *repeatable,* we mean that anyone should be able to re-create the experiment and achieve the same results.

Placebo controlled means that the treatment's effects are compared with the effects of taking placebo—a "treatment," such as a sugar pill, that is known to be medically ineffective. In placebo-controlled study, one group of subjects receives the medication being tested, while another group receives placebo.

People tend to feel better, often much better, when they believe they are receiving a treatment that might help them. This "placebo effect" can make a treatment seem effective even when it really does nothing on its own. A *double-blind* study eliminates the very powerful effects of suggestion by keeping the identity of the treatment and placebo groups secret from both patients and doctors. Thus both groups are "blind," and it is a "double-blind" study.

If the subjects knew whether they were receiving a treatment or placebo, they wouldn't respond to placebo. Likewise, if the researchers knew which group was receiving the treatment, they might give subtle, unintentional signs that they expected better results from the treatment group; or their own observations might be biased by their expectations. With a double-blind study, these influences of suggestion are canceled out.

> **When we say that an experiment is *repeatable,* we mean that anyone should be able to re-create the experiment and achieve the same results.**

An experiment is *randomized* when you use a random selection process to choose which people receive the active treatment, and which receive placebo. This way, you cannot bias the results by selecting certain people to receive the treatment whom you secretly believe might respond better.

Subjects Must Represent the General Population

In addition to these basic requirements, it is also important that the subjects of the study represent the general population. It wouldn't do, for example, to study a treatment's effects on a group of men, and then assume that the results would apply to women as well. (In fact, that mistake has been made many times!) As we shall see, the earliest feverfew study was flawed because it only enrolled people who already responded well to feverfew.

Mathematical Analysis

The outcome of the experiment also has to be analyzed mathematically to determine if the results are truly meaningful. In general, the more subjects there are in a study, the more likely it is that the results are valid for the population in general. If you flip a coin 20 times, and it comes up heads 14 times, it doesn't prove the coin is off balance. Though the laws of probability would predict heads coming up 10 times, a result of 14 is not unusual either. But if you flip the same coin 2,000 times, it would be very unusual to get heads 1,400 of those times. The first study's off-balanced result might just be due to chance; the second, larger study suggests strongly that the coin is rigged.

The more subjects there are in a study, the more likely it is that the results are valid for the population in general.

Likewise, you can't interpret the validity of a scientific study's findings without doing a statistical analysis that takes into account the size of the experiment and other factors. Statistical analysis can determine whether the results of an experiment of any size are due to chance or the treatment's actual effect.

Solving the Mystery

The investigation of an herb's potential medicinal use is not unlike unraveling a good murder mystery. For example, Sam Spade starts out with a set of observations gathered at the crime scene. He then organizes these observations to develop a theory, or suspicion, of how the murder was committed. Next he sets out to gather more facts to put his theory to the test. Once the investigation is completed and the detective feels his case is sound, he presents the case to a jury and the strength of the evidence is judged.

Statistical analysis can determine whether the results of an experiment of any size are due to chance or the treatment's actual effect.

Of course, fictional detectives like Sam Spade have one advantage scientists don't: Detectives can always pressure or coax the killer into making a confession that ties up all the loose ends in the story. For medical researchers, things aren't so easy. No matter how hard we work to get an herb like feverfew to give up its secrets, we know it will never really "talk"—instead, we will have to rely on a slow, laborious process of gathering clinical evidence, using the scientific method.

There have been three meaningful double-blind studies of feverfew. Unfortunately, the total number of subjects enrolled in these studies is still low. As we saw above, the larger the study, the more reliable the results.

The Difference Between
Anecdotal and Scientific Evidence

In our daily lives, we rely heavily on *anecdotal* evidence. For example, your best friend calls and says, "I've just tried this herb, feverfew, and my migraines are gone! You should take it." This is the kind of anecdotal evidence on which we often base our everyday decisions. You might decide to try the treatment that worked for your friend, just as you would choose the mechanic your cousin had a good experience with, or the restaurant that received five stars in a newspaper review.

However, when your best friend tells you that a certain treatment worked for her, it is hard to know for sure whether the treatment is actually the factor that made the difference. Even assuming that it was effective for your friend, you

When a drug is approved for use, it has usually been tested on about 1,000 to 2,000 individuals in double-blind placebo-controlled studies that continued for 4 to 6 weeks. To this point, 173 persons have taken part in studies of feverfew, in trials that have lasted many months. Although the length of the studies is satisfactory, the total number of subjects is still very small. Thus evidence for feverfew as a treatment for migraine is best described as "preliminary." Only when researchers conduct more and larger studies of feverfew will we know for certain whether or not this herb is an effective treatment for migraines.

still can't tell whether it would be effective for many other people, or for you, or whether the treatment is safe over the long term.

Doctors and medical researchers have learned to be wary of anecdotal evidence for medical treatments. Thanks to the power of suggestion—the "placebo effect" discussed in this chapter—virtually any substance can seem to be medically effective. Over the years, many treatments with a raft of testimonials (including some in wide use by physicians) have turned out to be no more effective than sugar pills. After they got caught wrong so many times, doctors finally decided to rely whenever possible only on evidence that comes from proper double-blind studies.

The London Study of Feverfew

Dr. E. Stewart Johnson, whom we met in chapter 1, conducted the first formal experiment on feverfew's effectiveness for migraine headaches. Following his initial success with his migraine patients, Dr. Johnson persuaded his colleagues to support formal research. He quickly enrolled 17 participants to take part in what is now called the London study of feverfew.[1]

Unfortunately, this 1985 trial did not meet all of the criteria for a proper scientific experiment. The main problem was that it recruited participants only from among people who were already using feverfew. This selection was a major flaw in the study. Maybe feverfew only works for a few people. Since everyone in the study was already using feverfew (presumably because it worked for them) the results might make feverfew look more widely effective than it really is. This kind of study flaw is called *self-selection.*

On the plus side, the study was placebo-controlled—the 17 participants were randomly assigned to either a group using feverfew or another that was given placebo. The study was also double-blind. Still, the total number of participants was small. The London study would be more conclusive if it had drawn on a larger group of subjects who were representative of the general population. Nevertheless, the results of the London study helped to shape future research questions and directly contributed to the later development of three well-designed feverfew experiments.

In the London study, the group receiving placebo soon developed a greater number of headaches and experienced more nausea and vomiting than the group receiving feverfew.

In this study all the participants were randomly assigned to either stay on feverfew or be switched without their knowledge to placebo for the 6 months of the study. The results were swift and dramatic. The group receiving placebo soon developed a greater number of headaches and experienced more nausea and vomiting than the group that was continuing to receive feverfew. At the start of the study, both groups had about the same average severity and frequency of headaches. By the end of the study, the placebo group was doing much worse than the feverfew group.

From this study, Dr. Johnson concluded that, for those persons currently taking feverfew and for whom the herb was an effective migraine prevention remedy, terminating the use of feverfew could result in increased migraines. However, this did not prove that the feverfew had effectively treated their migraines in the first place. It could be that feverfew users go through some kind of withdrawal when they stop taking feverfew. (This point will be discussed further in chapter 7.)

What Did We Learn?

The London study advanced our scientific knowledge, but not far enough. Although we now had a very strong suspicion that there was something about the herb feverfew that at least related to migraine symptoms, we didn't have proof. Like our fictional detective, medical science needed to move on from these initial observations. The next step was to see whether feverfew would be equally effective in a general population of people with migraines who were not self-selected.

The Nottingham Study

Word of Dr. Johnson's findings spread quickly through the British medical community. Many criticized his research methods and called for further research to substantiate his claims regarding feverfew and migraines. The more rigorously designed Nottingham study of 1988 was the result.[2]

This placebo-controlled double-blind study drew from a pool that was representative of adult individuals with migraines and recruited a much larger group—76 participants. The Nottingham study's results were published in a very highly regarded scientific journal, *The Lancet*.

The 76 participants were randomly divided into two groups. The first group was given feverfew for 4 months, and the second group was given placebo. After 4 months, the treatments were reversed: The first group was switched to placebo, and the second group was switched from the placebo to feverfew. This type of study is called a *crossover study*.

Dr. J. J. Murphy headed up the research team. Initially, Dr. Murphy and his colleagues held a public meeting to gather 190 people suffering from migraines, promising them the opportunity to participate in a new, experimental treatment for their migraines. To be eligible for the experiment, participants had to have suffered from migraines for at least 2 years and had to experience at least one migraine a month.

Participants of this experiment had to have suffered from migraines for at least 2 years and had to experience at least one migraine a month.

After the experiment had been explained, 76 of the 190 agreed to take part. A total of 23 had classic migraines and 53 had common migraines. There were 56 women and 20 men. Just over 23% of the participants had tried feverfew previously; almost two-thirds of this 23% had found it useful. Thus this pool of participants was much more representative of the general population than the London study's participants, 100% of whom were already using feverfew. (In Britain, feverfew is such a popular folk remedy that in any group of people with migraines you will find at least one person who uses it.)

At the start of the experiment, all the participants stopped taking any migraine-related drugs they had been using. During the first 4 months, participants kept a diary of migraine symptoms in which they wrote down the number and duration of each headache, the severity of each headache, and any associated symptoms. Participants were also asked to rate their headaches on a 10-point scale, with 1 being "the worst ever" and 10 being "the best ever." At the end of 4 months, the treatments for both groups were switched—the placebo group began to receive feverfew, and the feverfew group began to receive placebo instead—and the diaries were kept up for another 4 months. At the end of the second 4-month period, all the participants were asked if they had noticed any difference between the two 4-month treatments and, if so, which treatment they regarded as more effective.

By the end of the experiment, 17 participants had dropped out and 59 remained. Importantly, the individuals dropped out from both subgroups in roughly equal numbers—8 from one and 9 from the other—so the results were less affected by this than they might have been otherwise.

For the 59 participants who stayed throughout the 8-month experiment, there was a 24% decrease in the number of headaches during the period the participants were using feverfew. This difference (and all the others described here) was statistically significant. There was also a decrease in nausea and vomiting and duration and severity of headaches when they did occur.

Without knowing in which 4-month period they had received the feverfew, 59% of the participants identified the feverfew period as "more effective" and 24% chose the placebo period. The rest, 17%, said there was no difference. Feverfew reduced the number of headaches for people suffering classic migraines by 32%, and

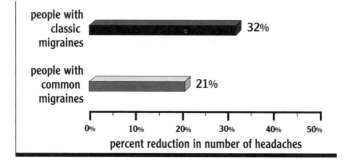

Figure 6. *Results from study indicate that feverfew can decrease the number of headaches* (Murphy, 1988)

for people suffering from common migraines by 21% (see figure 6).

Interestingly, mouth sores, the one side effect reported with the use of feverfew, actually occurred more often among those taking placebo than those taking the herb. No other significant side effects were reported.

What Did We Learn?

Dr. Murphy concluded that treatment with feverfew was clearly associated with a reduction in both migraine frequency and vomiting. In combination with the London study, the Nottingham study provided fairly strong evidence that feverfew was having some kind of a positive preventive effect on a large number of people with migraines.

Our fictional detective would now be proceeding with a bit more confidence, although still aware that he needed more evidence. At similar points in murder mystery novels, the detective often makes a faulty guess and pursues a suspect who turns out to be innocent. Research on feverfew took a similar wrong turn in 1996, when a Dutch study examined one of feverfew's major chemical ingredients, parthenolide, to see whether it was responsible for the herb's migraine-preventing effects.

Parthenolide

At the time of the Dutch study (discussed later in this chapter), a consensus had emerged that feverfew's antimigraine properties could probably be attributed to its parthenolide content.[3,4] As we discussed in chapter 1, the herb feverfew is rich in a family of compounds known as sesquiterpene lactones, primarily parthenolide. In test tube experiments, whole feverfew extracts have been shown to affect serotonin release (specifically from blood cells called platelets). Studies appeared to suggest that this effect was caused by parthenolide. Since serotonin release has been implicated in migraine headaches, parthenolide was the obvious suspect.

Both purified parthenolide and whole feverfew extracts have been found to decrease the synthesis of pain-producing substances within our bodies.

Furthermore, both purified parthenolide and whole feverfew extracts had been found to decrease the synthesis of prostaglandins, leukotrienes, and other pain-producing substances within our bodies. Parthenolide itself had also been found to interfere with both the contraction and relaxation of blood vessels.[5,6] All this information seemed to indicate that parthenolide was the active ingredient in feverfew.

Once parthenolide was identified as the likely suspect, investigators checked and found that different feverfew products available on the market varied widely in parthenolide content. In the interests of product quality, many herbal authorities subsequently called on the industry to standardize its products so that the daily dosage would supply about as much parthenolide as was in the feverfew used in the Nottingham study. Indeed, many indignant articles were written blasting manufacturers for selling "low-quality" feverfew that was low in parthenolide.

But everyone was jumping the gun. In retrospect, the evidence was never strong enough to support this conclusion. Parthenolide is apparently an innocent bystander, as the Dutch study showed.

The Dutch Study

A Dutch physician named Dr. C. De Weerdt was as much under the influence of the parthenolide concept as anyone else. Because he wasn't satisfied with the quality of the feverfew leaf available on the market, he sought to standardize a supply of feverfew based on its parthenolide content. Noting that the Nottingham study used 82 mg daily of whole, dried feverfew leaf containing 0.66% parthenolide, he and his fellow researchers made up a special alcoholic extract of feverfew that supplied the same amount of parthenolide daily. He used this special extract in the study, with high hopes that it was superior to what was available commercially. Unfortunately, it didn't work.

The experimental design of the Dutch study, like that of the Nottingham study, met the strict requirements of a rigorous scientific study. The study was placebo-controlled and double-blind, and the results were published in a respected scientific journal, *Phytomedicine*.[7] A total of 50 study participants were enrolled and randomly divided into two groups. One group was given feverfew for 4 months, followed by 4 months with placebo. The other group was given placebo for 4 months, followed by 4 months with feverfew. Given this study design, the experiment can be considered repeatable. The Dutch study must, therefore, be considered a well-designed scientific study, capable of yielding scientifically meaningful results.

The 50 study participants, including 42 women and 8 men, were recruited in the city of Emmen, Holland. All participants were adults who had suffered from migraines since their early youth. All of them suffered at least one migraine per month. At the start of the experiment, everyone was instructed to end his or her use of antimigraine medications. If necessary, however, participants were allowed to take medications that they had used in the past to quell an acute attack. As in the Nottingham study, participants were asked to keep headache diaries to record the frequency and severity of their headaches, along with other symptoms.

> **All participants were adults who had suffered from migraines since their early youth. All of them suffered at least one migraine per month.**

So, what happened? Very little. There was no significant difference between the two groups. Forty of the 50 participants completed the study. Some of the participants did better with feverfew than they did with the placebo, while others did better with the placebo. But, on average, there was no significant difference in the frequency or severity of migraine attacks in the two 4-month periods. The form of feverfew used in this study proved entirely ineffective. No one was more surprised than Dr. De Weerdt.

What Did We Learn?

As is often the case in both murder mysteries and medical research, failure can be as important as success. In the case of feverfew, the Dutch study established that feverfew's effect was not caused by parthenolide.

Apparently, there are other ingredients in whole feverfew leaf that are essential to its effectiveness. Although the alcohol extract contained plenty of parthenolide, many other components of the feverfew leaf were eliminated by the extractive process. For example, as Dr. De Weerdt pointed out in his research report, the amount of an oil called chrysanthenyl acetate was far lower in the Dutch preparation than in the whole leaf used in the Nottingham trial. Maybe this oil or other unidentified ingredients are necessary for feverfew to work. We simply do not know.

A shrewd detective would consider another possibility. Maybe the earlier trials were wrong, and feverfew was actually not effective in preventing migraines. After all, the studies that showed some effects were small and not completely conclusive. It has happened before that a few early, positive studies are contradicted by later trials.

But these negative results were soon followed by reports of positive results in another double-blind placebo-controlled study, one that tested a form of feverfew leaf similar to what was used in the Nottingham trial instead of an extract concentrated to its parthenolide content.

The Israeli Study

The Israeli study, like the London and Nottingham studies, used whole, dried feverfew leaf. It was published in a peer-reviewed, scientific journal, *Phytotherapy Research*.[8] The study drew from a general pool of people with migraines and recruited 57 participants, none of whom had ever used feverfew. (Feverfew is not as popular in Israel as in Britain, so it was easier to find people who'd never tried it.) The participants were randomly divided into two groups, one receiving feverfew and the other receiving placebo.

The 57 participants—47 women and 10 men—were chosen from among the patients in a hospital outpatient clinic. At the beginning of the study, all the participants recorded key information about their headaches, such as how intense their headaches generally were, how frequently they occurred, the nature of the head pain, and the severity of other symptoms, such as nausea or vomiting.

The study involved three phases. In the first phase, each group received two 50-mg capsules of feverfew a day for 60 days. In the second phase, the first group continued to receive feverfew for 30 days, while the second group was given placebo. In the third phase, these treatments were switched for the study's final 30 days. The form of feverfew used was similar to what was used in the London and Nottingham studies, although the growing conditions, geographic area, and species were all different. Dr. Palevitch used 50 mg of finely powdered feverfew leaves in gelatin capsules. The total parthenolide in a daily dose was 100 mg, compared with 0.5 mg in the Nottingham and Dutch studies.

The results of the Israeli study were strikingly positive. Interestingly, in this study feverfew decreased the intensity of migraine headaches (see figure 7). Unfortunately, the study did not report on whether there was any change in the frequency of migraines.

In the first phase, when all 57 participants used feverfew, the intensity of migraine headaches dropped

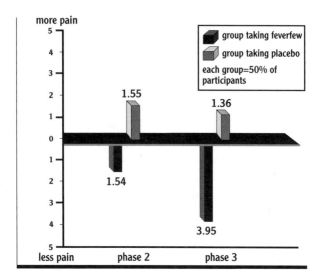

Figure 7. *Results from study show that pain intensity decreased in response to feverfew consumption* (Palevitch, 1997)

precipitously in both groups. There was a 10-point scale for pain, with 0 being no pain and 10 being the most severe pain. In the first phase, when both groups used feverfew, the pain fell in average by 4.27 points along the scale.

Feverfew significantly reduced headache pain, nausea, vomiting, and sensitivity to light.

In the second phase, the group continuing with feverfew had an average further drop of 1.54 points, and the group with placebo had an average rise of 1.55 points along the scale. In the third phase, the group that switched back to feverfew had an average drop of 3.95 points, where the group that switched to placebo had a rise of 1.36 points. Feverfew was also found to significantly reduce other symptoms such as nausea, vomiting, and sensitivity to light. There were no reported side effects in the Israeli study.

What Did We Learn?

Dr. Palevitch concluded, "The present clinical trial provides convincing evidence that consuming a feverfew leaf preparation can ease profoundly the pain intensity and the prevalence of the typical symptoms associated with migraine attacks."[9]

What Do These Studies Tell Us?

What do these four studies tell us? The London, Nottingham, and Israeli studies, taken together, strongly suggest that the whole feverfew leaf does something good for people with migraines. The Dutch study suggests that parthenolide alone probably isn't responsible for these effects.

To return to our murder mystery analogy, however, we're still a long way from the scene where the detective calls everyone into the study and dazzles them with the solution to the case. More research is needed to identify the active ingredient(s) in feverfew, and to further establish its effectiveness in preventing and/or relieving migraines.

This chapter began by raising three concerns with respect to the development of any new treatment: establishing its effectiveness, determining a form and dosage level, and finding that it did no harm. Based on the four studies discussed above, it appears likely that whole feverfew leaf can be effective for reducing either the number or the severity of migraine attacks for a large proportion of people suffering migraines. Feverfew also appears to be effective for reducing the severity of other migraine symptoms, such as nausea and vomiting. Feverfew does

An Accidental Cure

Elizabeth had suffered from migraines for nearly 20 years when, in her late 30s, she began to develop severe arthritis. A friend recommended that she try feverfew. While virtually no established scientific evidence supports the use of feverfew for arthritis, the folklore of its effectiveness persists—especially in Britain.

Elizabeth was an engineer by training, and she was reluctant to stray from conventional medical science. In fact, her sister had once suggested that she try feverfew for her migraines, but Elizabeth was happy with her conventional treatment, a beta-blocker that had reduced the frequency of her headaches down to one every 3 weeks or so. But conventional treatment wasn't helping her arthritis, which was interfering with her active outdoors life. So Elizabeth tried feverfew for her arthritis. At first, Elizabeth didn't see any improvement. (She continued to take the beta-blocker as well as the feverfew.)

After 2 months of daily usage, however, she began to notice a stark and unmistakable change, but not in her arthritis symptoms. Her migraines had all but disappeared. She had

not appear to cause significant side effects. While the whole leaf appears to be effective, an extract standardized to parthenolide content is not. Thus, while we have gone some way toward establishing the effectiveness and safety of feverfew, more, larger studies are needed before we can draw any firm conclusions.

one attack at the end of the second month, but it was the mildest attack she had ever had—no nausea, no vomiting, very mild head pain, and it lasted only 4 hours. Her usual migraine lasted about 10 hours and was often much longer. After 6 months on feverfew, Elizabeth's migraines were down to one very mild migraine attack every 3 months.

Elizabeth consulted with her doctor, who suggested Elizabeth stop taking the beta-blocker to see if the results would continue. They did. One year after she began taking feverfew, Elizabeth was off of her conventional antimigraine medication and she was down to one mild headache every 3 months. For Elizabeth, feverfew was a very successful treatment for migraines—it was more effective than the beta-blocker, and it had virtually no side effects.

Ironically, the feverfew never helped Elizabeth's arthritis, so she was forced to continue searching for an effective treatment for the problem that had prompted her to try feverfew in the first place. She eventually found help with glucosamine sulfate, but that is the subject of another book. (For more information on treatments for arthritis, see *The Natural Pharmacist Guide to Arthritis.*)

On the second question, we have further to go. We don't know what the active ingredient(s) in feverfew may be. However, feverfew is not alone in this. For most herbs on the market, the active ingredient remains unknown. This is even true of the best-documented herbs—St. John's wort, ginkgo, and saw palmetto. Based on the results of many double-blind trials, we are fairly certain that they are effective—but we don't know for sure what chemicals in them make them work.

Actually, it is hard to think of more than a handful of medicinal herbs for which we conclusively know the active ingredient. One reason is that herbs, unlike drugs, are made up of thousands of chemical constituents. Another reason is that once an active ingredient is discovered, it is generally turned into a drug, and the herb stops being used.

For a complete discussion of new treatments and whether or not they're harmful, see chapter 7.

How Does Feverfew Work?

We don't know how feverfew works for migraines. This is an important question for research to address. At this point, all we can do is make reasonable guesses based on limited information. We can be reasonably certain that parthenolide alone is not the basis for feverfew's effectiveness. But it may be that parthenolide is partly responsible, in combination with other unknown compounds that were missing from the Dutch study's feverfew extract.

Studies have found that purified parthenolide can decrease the synthesis of prostaglandins, leukotrienes, and other pain-producing substances within the body and can interfere with both the contraction and relaxation of blood vessels. As mentioned above, the substance chrysanthenyl acetate might also contribute to feverfew's antimigraine success. In addition, feverfew contains several chemicals called hydrophobic flavonols, which have recently been getting attention as possible anti-inflammatory agents.[10]

All of these findings point us toward a range of intriguing possibilities. For now, however, we are just at the stage of formulating a hypothesis. We cannot say with any certainty what may or may not be the true basis for feverfew's success.

Dr. Varro Tyler, a well-known herbal expert, has this to say about feverfew and medicinal herbs in general: "While we may as yet be unable to isolate, purify, and market a botanical's chemical constituent for use as a drug, the herb that contains it may still be used in its natural or phytomedicinal form and desirable therapeutic effects may be achieved."[11]

With feverfew, we have discovered enough to justify curiosity and excitement. But we can't yet explain what happens in your body when you take feverfew. The case remains open.

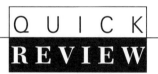

QUICK REVIEW

- We need to answer three questions about feverfew as a treatment for migraines: (1) Is it effective? (2) How should it be taken? (3) Is it safe?

- Medical science has devised a standard experimental procedure with four elements to validate the results of experiments. The experiments must be *repeatable, placebo-controlled, double-blind,* and *randomized.* To date, three studies of feverfew as a treatment for migraines have met these requirements. In addition, there has been one study that provided limited but still useful information.

- The cumulative evidence from three valid studies suggests that feverfew leaf is indeed an effective preventive treatment for migraines. It appears to decrease the frequency and severity of migraine attacks, as well as accompanying symptoms such as nausea and vomiting.

- It was previously thought that the substance parthenolide was the active ingredient in feverfew. However, a study that showed zero effect from a feverfew extract standardized to parthenolide content has shattered this faith. Apparently feverfew leaf has other important ingredients in it besides parthenolide.

- We don't know yet how feverfew works in the body, or what its active ingredient(s) may be. Chapter 7 will address research on feverfew's safety.

How to Take Feverfew

N ow that you've read about what feverfew can do, you might be ready to try it. This chapter tells you what is known about the dosage and proper form of feverfew, and what to expect when you take it.

Dosage

We don't really know the ideal dosage of feverfew. In the Nottingham study, participants took 82 mg of dried encapsulated leaf daily, while the Israeli study used 100 mg a day of leaf. It probably makes sense to take the same overall dosage of dried feverfew leaf: in the range of 80 to 100 mg per day.

What's the Best Form of Feverfew to Take?

In England, many people grow their own feverfew and chew on the fresh, raw leaves as a home remedy for migraine headaches. This is certainly the most natural way to use feverfew! However, as we will see in chapter 7, chewing feverfew leaf can cause mouth sores in some people. Also, many people in the United States prefer to take a convenient capsule.

There is always a concern that dried herb may be less effective than fresh because of the processing steps involved. However, in the Nottingham and Israeli studies, participants used encapsulated, dried feverfew leaf, and it was successful. This is the form of feverfew most commonly used today.

The capsules should be made with as few processing steps as possible and used quickly after manufacture. Ideally, we would use feverfew that was identical in all respects to the feverfew used in the Nottingham or Israeli studies. Since this is not a practical possibility, trial and error may be required before you find a source of feverfew that works for you. The most reliable guide to a quality herbal product is an herbalist, pharmacist, or other health practitioner who prescribes herbs.

The most reliable guide to herbal products is an herbalist, pharmacist, or other health practitioner who is knowledgeable in herbs.

Some feverfew products will state a certain percentage of parthenolide. However, as I discussed in chapter 6, parthenolide is no longer believed to be the active ingredient in feverfew. Still, it may make sense to purchase feverfew leaf products that contain 0.2 to 0.66% parthenolide, since that was the percentage used in the Nottingham and Dutch studies, and this may mean that the leaf is somewhat similar in makeup. But make sure you are getting feverfew leaf, and not extract, as extracts concentrated to parthenolide content may not be effective.

Where Can You Find Feverfew?

Feverfew isn't hard to find today. Your local pharmacy probably has a section for "natural remedies," and many cities and towns today have a local herbal store as well. Grocery stores that specialize in "natural" foods usually carry herbs as well. You can also grow it in your garden, and in parts of eastern North America—roughly from Quebec· to Maryland, and west to Ohio—feverfew can also be found growing wild. If you're lucky, maybe you'll meet someone who can show you how to identify it. But don't try to collect it in the wild unless you know what you are doing. It can be hard to tell plants apart, and you might take something poisonous by mistake. I recommend foraging for feverfew in a pharmacy or other store instead.

Feverfew is best used as a preventive treatment. This means that you should follow a sustained, consistent regimen. To be effective, feverfew should be taken every day.

When Should You Take Feverfew?

Feverfew is best used as a preventive treatment for migraines. This means that you should follow a sustained, consistent regimen. To be effective, feverfew should be taken every day.

Meg's Story

When it came to feverfew, Meg was a skeptic. She had been a practicing pharmacist for nearly 20 years. Over that time, many of her clients had come to her with a range of questions about this or that new "breakthrough" herb that seemed to be all the rage for a while and then quietly faded from view. As a pharmacist, Meg wasn't easily swayed by hype; she wanted to see the research before she formed any opinions about a new herbal treatment.

When she started hearing about feverfew, though, Meg was interested, since she suffered from migraines herself. From her clients' as well as her own experience, she knew about the struggle to find an effective treatment with a manageable level of side effects. She herself had recently switched from beta-blockers, which were only marginally effective for her, to sumatriptan. The sumatriptan worked for her, but she didn't like taking it as often as her frequent headaches required.

One of Meg's clients who had suffered from migraines all her life had just returned from a trip to visit her family in England and was surprised to hear from their local doctor

It doesn't seem to matter whether you take feverfew early or late in the day. It also doesn't seem to matter whether you divide the dosage in half and take the herb twice a day rather than all at once. Your own personal habits can dictate this process. Many people prefer to take feverfew with meals, both because it's easier to remember that way and also because, as with all medicines, there is that many people in her family's town used feverfew for migraines.

When Meg heard this story, her interest was piqued. She read up on the London and the Nottingham studies (this was before the Dutch and Israeli studies had been published) and finally decided to try it herself. Within a couple of months, she began to see differences. Both the frequency and the severity of her migraines subsided.

Made enthusiastic by her success, Meg became more willing to support her clients who wanted to try feverfew. She always made sure to explain that the scientific findings were not yet conclusive and warned prospective users of feverfew's potential dangers for pregnant women and those taking certain medications. Nonetheless, at least 40 people purchased feverfew over a 1-year period.

In order to roughly gauge the herb's effectiveness, Meg asked her clients who used feverfew to keep her informed of their progress. While this was not a fully scientific approach, her "unscientific poll" found that feverfew seemed to be significantly effective in about half of those who tried it .

a slight chance that the feverfew leaf will mildly irritate your stomach.

Some people report that taking a high dose of feverfew (2 to 5 times the usual recommended daily amount, or 160 to 500 mg) at the onset of a headache can abort an attack. Others say that taking moderately high doses of feverfew (2 times the usual daily dosage, or 160 to

200 mg) throughout a migraine instead of at the onset can reduce symptoms and reduce the duration of the headache. However, we don't have any scientific evidence to tell us whether this method works, or even if it is safe. (See chapter 7 for a discussion of feverfew's safety.)

Who Should Not Take Feverfew?

Because it is generally taken on a continuous basis, feverfew is most appropriate for people who have frequent migraine headaches. Feverfew is probably not worth taking every day for people who only get migraines once or twice a year. Generally, feverfew only begins to be practical for those who experience migraines at least once a month.

Trisha's and Marilyn's experiences with feverfew illustrate this point. Trisha generally had one migraine attack every 3 or 4 months, while Marilyn suffered through at least two attacks a week. The two were friends, and both decided to try feverfew after hearing about it on a radio program. Each took the same daily dosage of 80 mg of feverfew each morning. Marilyn noticed an immediate improvement. Her twice-weekly headaches dropped in frequency to about once or twice a month, and when she did get a migraine it wasn't very severe. She was very happy to stick with the daily routine of taking feverfew, given such excellent results.

For Trisha, on the other hand, the benefits were less clear. After 2 months of taking feverfew, she hadn't had any headaches. But since her headaches usually came only several times a year, this was no big surprise. After a couple of months, she started forgetting to take her feverfew. When she finally did have a migraine, she again took feverfew religiously for a while, but then her attention lapsed again.

Marilyn forgot to take her feverfew from time to time as well. However, in her case, each lapse was followed by a return to her old pattern of frequent migraines. She had every incentive to continue, while Trisha did not. Trisha eventually quit entirely, which was probably sensible. It doesn't really make sense to take feverfew daily to prevent migraines that don't come very often anyway.

Furthermore, before you decide to use feverfew for your migraines, you should consult your doctor. Migraine symptoms can be the first sign of other serious illnesses that may require specific treatment. You don't want to treat a brain tumor with feverfew, for example. (Keep in mind, however, that brain tumors are very rare.)

There are also certain safety issues associated with feverfew. For example, pregnant women or those taking anticoagulants such as Coumadin should stay away from the herb. Chapter 7 will discuss all these safety issues in detail.

Before using feverfew for your migraines, you should consult your doctor. Migraine symptoms can be the first sign of other serious illnesses that may require treatment.

What to Expect from Treatment

According to the research described in the previous chapter, feverfew appears to be able to reduce the frequency of migraine headaches, as well as reduce the severity of nausea, light sensitivity, and pain during an attack. Benefits usually develop fairly rapidly, but full effects may take weeks to develop.

> **If feverfew works for you, it might be a better alternative than other available treatments.**

One big advantage of feverfew is that it causes practically no side effects. If feverfew works for you, it might be a better alternative than other available treatments. But there is no way to predict in advance whether or not it will help.

Putting it all together, feverfew can be described as a useful and safe treatment—not a miracle cure, but an option that many people with migraines may deeply appreciate.

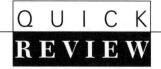

QUICK REVIEW

- We don't as yet know the best form or the ideal dosage of feverfew. The usual advice at present is to take the same amount used in the successful studies of feverfew, 80 to 100 mg daily of dried feverfew leaf in capsule form.

- It may be a good idea to get feverfew containing 0.2% to 0.66% parthenolide in order to duplicate the leaf used in the Nottingham and Dutch studies. However, since parthenolide is no longer believed to be the active ingredient, I don't recommend using feverfew extracts standardized to parthenolide content.

- Feverfew seems to be most effective when it's taken daily to prevent migraines.

- There hasn't been any research to establish whether or not feverfew is effective for treating the pain of a headache once it's started, although it is sometimes used for that purpose.

Safety Issues

As we have seen, feverfew seems to be an effective treatment for many people with migraines who try it. Although we need more research before we can draw firm conclusions about feverfew's effectiveness or the proper dosage to use, we do have some scientific evidence to guide us. This chapter will address the next important question: Is feverfew safe?

What Is "Safe"?

Medical doctors aim to meet the high standard of the Hippocratic oath: First, do no harm. In many ways, this oath has also been the rallying cry for advocates of natural medicine as well. One of the main reasons for the interest in herbal medicines today is that most common medicinal herbs are less toxic on average than most drugs, and they also tend to produce fewer side effects than pharmaceuticals. However, it is important to realize that "natural" is not a guarantee of safety. Many "natural" substances can be dangerous, and it is never wise to take an herbal medicine without the advice of a doctor or other knowledgeable health professional.

This chapter will describe what we know about feverfew's safety. For any medicine, safety is a matter of two things: side effects and toxicity. *Side effects* are unwanted physical effects that occur during normal use. They usually aren't dangerous, but they can be unpleasant or disruptive. *Toxicity* is the medicine's potential to be poisonous when taken in excess. In general, as we will see, feverfew seems to have very few side effects and low toxicity. These results are not surprising, since we know that feverfew has been used as a folk medicine in England for decades or longer without any reports of poisoning or serious side effects.

Many "natural" substances can be dangerous, and it is never wise to take an herbal medicine without the advice of a doctor or other knowledgeable health professional.

Yet it's important to realize that feverfew's safety has not yet been thoroughly studied. There have been only four clinical trials, involving a relatively small total number of participants, and none extended for longer than a few months. It's possible that there are side effects that simply haven't come to light yet. We also don't know whether feverfew presents any special risks when combined with other medications.

Feverfew's Excellent Side-Effect Profile

The research to date on feverfew has found practically no side effects. In the three major studies of feverfew, neither encapsulated dried feverfew nor feverfew extract caused more side effects than placebo. (It's a surprising fact, but true, that people report all kinds of side effects from placebo treatment. You have to take this "background noise" into account when looking at the side-effect rates caused by a treatment.)

Only the tiny London study found any significant problems. In that study, which used raw feverfew leaf, 11.3% of the participants reported that they developed mouth sores and/or tongue irritation. However, this problem seems to be confined to people who chew their feverfew. Feverfew in capsule form apparently does not cause mouth sores. Some of the participants

The research to date on feverfew has found practically no side effects.

in the Nottingham study, which used a capsule form of feverfew, did report mouth sores—but there were more reports of mouth sores among the placebo group than among the participants who were taking feverfew!

Sores in the mouth simply happen from time to time. But it is probably fair to say that unless you chew feverfew leaf, the herb will not cause this problem. Mild digestive distress was also seen in some participants in the London study. However, no similar gastrointestinal side effects were reported in any of the other three studies discussed in chapter 5.[1]

Thus there is some weak evidence that chewing dried feverfew leaf may be associated with the side effects of mouth sores and mild gastrointestinal distress. I recommend you take feverfew in capsule form to avoid these potential problems.

Is There Such a Thing As Post-Feverfew Syndrome?

In the London study, as you might remember from chapter 5, all of the study's participants were already taking feverfew with some success before the study began.[2] The placebo group showed a dramatic increase in headache severity and other symptoms as soon as they stopped taking feverfew. One participant in this group also experienced a number of symptoms that, Dr. Johnson theorized, might be caused by withdrawal from feverfew. These symptoms—including not only headache but also insomnia, nervousness, and discomfort in the joints—raise the question of whether there might be a "post-feverfew syndrome" in some people when they stop taking feverfew.

However, aside from this one report, no "post-feverfew syndrome" was found in any of the feverfew studies, including the crossover studies in which the group that was initially given feverfew was later switched to placebo. If "post-feverfew syndrome" was common, it should have appeared in the crossover studies.

The weight of clinical evidence to date suggests that the phenomenon of "post-feverfew

Dr. Steven Bratman notes that, among his patients, "no one has ever showed signs of withdrawal when they stopped taking feverfew."

syndrome" is at most an extremely rare occurrence. Dr. Steven Bratman notes that he has prescribed feverfew for about 100 individuals during the past several years. "No one has ever showed signs of withdrawal when they stopped taking it," he says.

Based on the current research as well as what we can deduce from feverfew's popularity as a folk medicine in England, feverfew seems to have few or no side effects.

Comparing Feverfew's Side Effects with Side Effects of Conventional Antimigraine Medications

In chapter 4, we saw that there are four categories of conventional antimigraine medications that, like feverfew, can *prevent* migraines: beta-blockers, ergot drugs, calcium channel–blockers, and antidepressants. Because all these drugs cause a significant number of side effects, feverfew seems to offer a significant potential advantage.

Beta-blockers and ergot drugs are the two most popular forms of conventional migraine prevention medications. As we saw in chapter 3, the side effects associated with the use of beta-blockers include fatigue, depression, impotence, worsened asthma, reduced blood pressure, a lowered pulse rate, dizziness, weight gain, gastrointestinal symptoms, cold hands and feet, and nightmares. For ergot drugs,

Because all these preventive conventional drugs cause a significant number of side effects, feverfew seems to offer a significant potential advantage.

the list is shorter, but also potentially troublesome: nausea, muscle cramps, abdominal pain, problems with blood circulation, weight gain, and leg cramps.

The side effects associated with the use of calcium channel–blockers include constipation, fluid retention, drowsiness, cardiac dysfunction, and in some cases, headaches. The main type of antidepressant used for migraine prevention is the selective serotonin-reuptake inhibitors (SSRIs). The side effects associated with SSRIs include nausea, insomnia, sexual disturbances (impotence in men and inability to achieve orgasm in women), and mild agitation or nervousness.

On the basis of side effects, feverfew looks pretty good compared to these options! Presuming it works for you, it may be much more pleasant to use than standard migraine prevention drugs. However, with drugs there is a much greater opportunity to discover side effects. Not only are they tested in large-scale studies, but after a drug comes on the market there is a formal reporting process that records harm occurring even as rarely as in one case in a million. There is no such reporting process for herbs in the United States. (There is one in Germany, but it is not as stringent as standard systems for reporting adverse reactions to drugs.)

Although there are no reports of severe adverse effects due to feverfew, we can't consider it as absolutely proven to be safe.

Therefore, although there are no reports of severe adverse effects due to feverfew, we can't consider it as absolutely proven to be safe. It is possible that future research will discover some hitherto unrecognized problem.

But at present, it certainly seems likely that feverfew causes significantly fewer side effects than standard conventional treatments.

Toxicity

Side effects generally go away when you stop using whatever caused them, and they occur at normal or even low dosages of a treatment. We usually use a different word, *toxicity,* to refer to more serious adverse effects including actual injury to the body. Most commonly, toxic reactions occur when a substance is taken in excessive dosages.

A medicine can have few side effects but high toxicity, and vice versa. For example, acetaminophen hardly ever causes any side effects; but if you take more than the recommended amount, your liver can be damaged, and a large overdose can be fatal. Conversely, Prozac causes many side effects, but massive overdoses generally cause little more than a bad stomachache.

The usual procedure for studying toxicity is to experiment on animals such as rats and mice. Typically, researchers give progressively higher dosages to animals until the dosage is high enough to kill half the animals. (Most substances, including salt, are toxic if they are given in massively high dosages.) This dosage is then reported as the LD_{50}, or lethal dosage in 50% of the animals. To adjust for the size of the animal, this dosage is usually stated in proportion to body weight. A related procedure is to give the substance to pregnant animals and then look for birth defects.

Feverfew has been tested in such a fashion. Its toxicity is so low that researchers were unable to find an LD_{50} dosage. When guinea pigs and rats were given 150 and 100 times the human dosage, respectively, there were no adverse effects on the animals.[3]

Beverly's Story

Beverly was a 23-year-old math teacher who had suffered from migraines for 4 years. She started treating them with the prescription drug dihydroergotamine (DHE-45) for relief. At first she responded well, but over time DHE-45 started to fail, and the attacks grew more severe and frequent than they had been at the beginning.

Beverly's headaches generally began in the morning, causing tremendous pain with severe nausea and vomiting. She could do nothing but lie in a dark room far from noise. Her doctor switched her to sumatriptan (Imitrex), but the results weren't much better. Eventually, Beverly was switched to a beta-blocker, Corgard, to try to prevent migraines before they started.

At first, the beta-blocker worked quite well. Beverly went from having 2 to 3 migraines a week to having no more than 1 every 2 months. Though the severity of her attacks also seemed to wane, Beverly experienced uncomfortable side effects from the beta-blocker, including fatigue so pervasive that she thought her debilitating migraines might be better.

She also experienced bouts of depression, for which she needed treatment with Prozac. Switching beta-blockers, from Corgard to Inderal, did not improve matters. Her side effects

Another study addressed the question of whether feverfew causes chromosome or DNA damage. Thirty women with migraines who had taken feverfew for 11 months or longer were compared to a similar group of individuals who had not taken feverfew.[4] No difference was continued, and she started to feel more fear of her medication than of the migraines themselves.

One evening, a guest speaker at Beverly's migraine support group gave a presentation on feverfew. The speaker explained that feverfew had a long history of use and was very popular in Europe, especially in England. Most intriguing of all to Beverly was feverfew's lack of side effects. Soon, she purchased some feverfew and started taking one 82-mg capsule every 24 hours. At the same time, under the supervision of her physician, she stopped taking beta-blockers, to avoid the side effects, and went back to sumatriptan for relief as needed.

In the first month of her new regime of feverfew plus the occasional use of sumatriptan, Beverly suffered two fairly severe migraines. In the second month, for the first time in nearly 4 years, she had no headache. In the third month, she had one relatively mild migraine attack with no nausea or vomiting. Over the next 2 years, her migraine attacks settled down to 1 fairly mild migraine every 3 months. She seldom uses sumatriptan anymore.

(continues)

found between the two groups, suggesting (but not proving) that feverfew is not likely to cause cancer or birth defects.

Additional evidence for the safety of feverfew came from the studies we saw in chapter 4 that evaluated the

Beverly's Story *(continued)*

For Beverly, feverfew turned out to be just the answer she was looking for. It had none of the beta-blockers' terrible side effects, and it turned out to be even more effective. Even if the feverfew hadn't proven to be quite so effective for her, Beverly might have still preferred it to the beta-blockers because of its lack of side effects. We really need more research to find out just how many people could benefit from feverfew, precisely how it compares in effectiveness to standard medications, and whether it offers any hidden risks.

herb's effectiveness. In these studies, the researchers also measured key biochemical changes in the bodies of the study participants. All the participants were given a battery of physical tests (including measures of key body chemicals, blood counts, and urinalysis) before and after the study. In the end, the use of feverfew was not associated with significant changes in any of these key indicators.

Putting all this information together, it is safe to say that feverfew appears to be a fairly nontoxic substance.

Drug Interactions

In general, most widely used medicinal herbs appear to be relatively nontoxic and to produce few side effects. However, herb–drug interactions—that is, the unintended effects when a medicinal herb is combined with a drug—are another issue. Although little is known about herb–drug interactions in general, it appears very likely that they may occur. After all, both herbs and drugs interact with your body, often in similar ways.

Many complications can be imagined. An herb might diminish the activity of a drug, increase its activity, cause it to be metabolized more quickly or more slowly, or either interfere with or enhance its excretion. Unfortunately, very little research is available on herb–drug interactions. We usually find out about such interactions more or less by accident—if an interaction happens and a doctor notices it and publishes a report.

There are no known drug interactions involving feverfew. However, there is reason to be concerned that feverfew might enhance the effects of drugs that "thin" the blood, such as warfarin (Coumadin), heparin, and aspirin. Some of feverfew's chemical constituents are known to affect the activity of platelets, which play a major role in blood clotting. It is quite possible that if feverfew is combined with drugs that produce a similar effect, there might be an increased risk of serious bleeding. No such effect has ever been observed, but since we don't know whether or not it's possible, it is best to be cautious.

Though there are no known drug interactions involving feverfew, there is reason to be concerned that feverfew might enhance the effects of drugs that "thin" the blood.

However, the results of one study failed to bear out this concern. A group of 10 people who had taken feverfew for many years were compared with 4 similar people who had stopped feverfew 6 months earlier.[5] No differences were found in the platelet functions of the two groups.

Still, medications might amplify small differences in platelet function, so it pays to be cautious.

Long-Term Safety

Long-term safety is very difficult to determine for any treatment, whether herb or drug. It's true that feverfew has been used for many centuries. However, if side effects take a long time to develop, and only occur in a relatively small percentage of people, it would be very hard for traditional herbalists to recognize the connection. Suppose, for example, that taking a certain herb increased your risk for cancer very slightly—maybe 1%—and only after about 20 years. Neither the herbalist nor the patient would be likely to consider that the cancer was even partly caused by the herb taken so long ago.

Actually, the same problem happens with drugs. Unless you continue a placebo-controlled study of a large number of subjects for many years, you can't be certain about long-term effects. Needless to say, very few studies can be continued for such a length of time. With feverfew, the longest-running studies were 8 months—4 for treatment and 4 for follow-up. (Many drugs on the market have not been studied even this long.) It is quite possible that many drugs and herbs cause a certain incidence of unidentified long-term consequences.

An easier way to find long-term problems is to compare the health of people who have taken a certain treatment for a long time with that of other people, similar in other respects, who have not taken the treatment. This method is less reliable than a placebo-controlled study because there might be many unrecognized differences between the two groups. But such studies can still be useful. Unfortunately, none have been done for feverfew (or for many other herbs and drugs).

Thus we can't say for certain that feverfew is safe to use in the long term. In this, feverfew is in very good company. We could say the same for many drugs in use today.

We *can* say, however, that no long-term health risks associated with feverfew have come to light so far.

On the other hand, as we saw in chapter 4, there is definite evidence of long-term risk for some antimigraine drugs. For example, methysergide has been associated with the development of fibrous tissue that can impair the function of the lungs, circulatory system, and kidneys.

No long-term health risks associated with feverfew have come to light so far.

Is Feverfew Safe During Pregnancy?

Perhaps the most serious safety concerns regarding feverfew have to do with its potential effects on pregnant women. Historically, feverfew has been used to induce childbirth or to cause abortions. Although there is no modern clinical evidence that feverfew could disrupt a pregnancy, pregnant women should avoid using feverfew just to be on the safe side. Your doctor should be able to help you evaluate your options for migraine prevention and relief during pregnancy.

Is Feverfew Safe for Children?

Another important safety consideration for any medication is whether or not it is safe for children to take. Children's bodies in their various stages of development may react differently than adults' bodies. Unfortunately, there is almost no scientific evidence relating to the safety of feverfew as a migraine treatment for children. Of the four studies considered in chapter 5, only the Israeli study

Barbara's Story

Barbara was a 30-year-old single mom working as a secretary. For almost 15 years she had fought off an average of at least one migraine headache per month. She had been prescribed Inderal, a beta-blocker, but it did not work perfectly and it made her feel sleepy.

When sumatriptan came on the market, it was a great step forward for Barbara, reducing her migraines to a manageable nuisance. Under her doctor's supervision, she quit Inderal without any ill effect.

However, after a couple of years Barbara became uncomfortable with the notion of relying on sumatriptan to quell her pain. She preferred natural treatments over chemical solutions whenever possible. Barbara had heard about developments in the field of alternative medicine, and she decided she wanted to try an herbal medicine.

Barbara happened to live in one of the handful of states that licensed naturopathic practitioners to be primary care providers. Her naturopathic physician advised her against immediately dropping sumatriptan to relieve her migraine symptoms. Rather, he suggested that Barbara keep using the drug

included participants under 18, and that study did not attempt to identify safety issues specifically for children.

For this reason, it is especially important that a doctor or other qualified health professional oversee any use of feverfew to prevent migraines in a child. It is also as needed and begin taking daily doses of feverfew to help prevent future migraines.

After 2 months of taking feverfew, Barbara did not notice any improvement. Her headaches were just as frequent and just as severe. She continued to take her sumatriptan for relief, and though she was beginning to seriously question all the hype she'd heard about natural medicine, she also kept taking the feverfew.

After 4 months, Barbara began to discern some changes. Her headaches were just as frequent, but they were significantly less severe. During one migraine attack, she did not even need sumatriptan for relief. A single Tylenol did the trick.

After 6 months, for the first time in 15 years, Barbara had gone 2 months without a headache. The headache she later experienced was extremely mild. Before long, she had reduced her chronic migraine condition to one mild attack every 4 months. She hadn't needed her sumatriptan in months.

Interestingly, in Barbara's case feverfew took a long time to reach full effect, longer than the duration of most of the studies involving feverfew. Barbara's experience suggests that longer-term studies should be done.

worth noting that the effectiveness of feverfew for children with migraines has not been documented. There are no studies that specifically measure the effectiveness of feverfew for the prevention of migraines in children. The use of feverfew by children can, therefore, neither be recommended nor discouraged based on the available research.

Is Feverfew Safe for Those with Liver or Kidney Disease?

The body processes foreign substances by excreting them through the kidneys, by metabolizing them in the liver, or both. In people with severe diseases of the liver or kidneys, this natural ability may be hampered. Many otherwise safe or reasonably safe drugs become more dangerous when they are given to people with such conditions. Although feverfew has not been definitely shown to be harmful in those with liver or kidney disease, as a matter of prudence such individuals should only take feverfew under medical supervision.

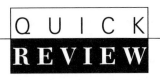

QUICK
REVIEW

- The safety of an herb involves two things: *side effects* and *toxicity.*
- In general, feverfew seems to be almost free of side effects and to have very low toxicity.
- The only side effects found in the research on feverfew so far include sores in the mouth, irritation of the tongue, and mild gastrointestinal distress. All of these side effects were found in a single study, in which participants chewed dried feverfew leaf. Feverfew in capsule or extract form does not seem to cause these problems.

- One study reported an individual who experienced what might have been "post-feverfew syndrome," or a withdrawal reaction after the person's feverfew was replaced with placebo. However, none of the larger studies on feverfew's effectiveness have found withdrawal reactions.

- Toxicity studies using animals found no signs of toxicity with feverfew, even at 100 or 150 times the human dosage.

- Feverfew is not known to interact dangerously with any conventional drugs. However, because feverfew might affect platelet activity, do not combine feverfew with drugs or herbs that thin the blood, except on medical advice.

- Pregnant women should not take feverfew because the herb's traditional use to induce labor and abortions suggests that it might interfere with a pregnancy.

- The safety of feverfew for children, nursing mothers, or those with severe liver or kidney disease has not been established.

Other Alternative Treatments for Migraines

B esides feverfew, there are other alternative therapies for migraines that you should know about. This chapter will describe four alternative therapies that are currently popular for migraines: magnesium, 5-HTP, acupuncture, and fish oil. As we will see, all four of these treatments need to be studied further, but initial research is promising. Please note that all these treatments are used primarily to prevent migraines, not to relieve the pain of a migraine after it's started.

Magnesium: Promising for Preventing Migraines

As we saw in chapter 3, there is a link between the body's magnesium levels and the physiological mechanisms that underlie a migraine attack. One long-held theory suggests that a magnesium deficiency might predispose a person to suffer from migraines.

A 1995 study compared a group of people with migraines and a similar group of people who did not have migraines. The results showed that the people with migraines were significantly more likely to have low levels of magnesium in their red blood cells than people without migraines.[1] Red blood cell magnesium levels are sometimes used to indicate the amount of magnesium in the body as a whole.

In another study, medical researchers measured magnesium levels in the brains of people with migraines during an attack and found that the magnesium levels were lower than in the brains of otherwise similar people who did not have migraines.[2]

Magnesium is known to influence the dilation and constriction of blood vessels. In addition, changes in magnesium levels have been associated with other features of migraines, including the spreading alteration of electrical activity in the brain that occurs during migraine headaches and the release of neurotransmitters.[3,4] As we saw in chapter 3, all these physiological changes are associated with a migraine attack.

For all these reasons, it has long been suspected that magnesium supplementation might play a useful role in migraine prevention. However, the evidence I've mentioned thus far is indirect. None of it really proves that if you take magnesium your headaches will improve. To find that out, we really need direct studies in which people with migraines are actually given magnesium, and compared with a control group not given magnesium. This type of research is still in its infancy.

What Is the Scientific Evidence for Magnesium?

A recent, double-blind placebo-controlled trial enrolled 81 people with frequent migraines (an average of 3.6 per month) and followed them for 12 weeks.[5] Half received a daily dose of 600 mg of magnesium, while the other half received placebo.

The results showed that between weeks 9 and 12 the participants taking the magnesium had a 41.6% decrease in the frequency of their migraines and a reduced need for medication. The participants receiving placebo also saw a reduction in the frequency of their headaches, but only by 15.8%. This difference was statistically significant. (See figure 8 for results of magnesium.) The only observed side effects with magnesium were diarrhea (18.6% of participants) and digestive irritation (4.7% of participants).

Good results have also been seen in other small studies.[6,7] One enrolled 20 women who suffered menstrual migraines. This study was a 4-month, double-blind placebo-controlled trial. The treatment group was given a daily dose of 360 mg of magnesium per day, and the other group was given placebo. The group receiving magnesium reported that both the intensity and duration of their headaches decreased. The placebo group had no significant improvement. While these findings are promising, the number of participants (20) was too small to result in statistically meaningful findings.[8]

> **The research on magnesium is in its early stages. What can be said is that preliminary evidence appears to be more positive than negative.**

One study did not find magnesium helpful.[9] However, its design has been criticized on various grounds, including that it used criteria for improvement so strict that few standard migraine drugs would have been found effective either.[10] Still, it is fair to say that the research on magnesium is in its early stages.

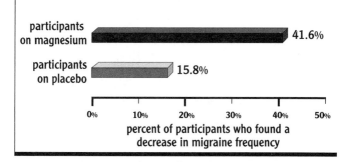

Figure 8. *Results of study show that magnesium reduces frequency of migraine headaches* (Mazzota, 1995)

The most that can be said at present is that preliminary evidence appears to be more positive than negative.

Dosage

Based on the positive studies noted above, a reasonable daily dosage of magnesium supplements to prevent migraine attacks is from 360 to 600 mg per day, as magnesium citrate. Other forms of magnesium may be acceptable as well.

By comparison, the recommended daily allowance for nutritional purposes in adults ranges from 250 to 400 mg. Since magnesium deficiency is common in Americans, supplementation is probably a generally healthful step anyway.

Calcium intake can interfere with magnesium absorption, so you might want to take your calcium and magnesium pills separately. The body needs vitamin B_6 to use magnesium properly, and B_6 deficiency is also common, so taking that vitamin as well may be useful.

Safety Issues

The dosages of magnesium used in treatment are not far above the recommended daily allowance of this mineral

Ted's Story

Ted first developed migraines at age 27. He was an auto mechanic who spent most of his day underneath cars, with a loud chorus of power tools blasting away in the background. His migraine attacks were not severe, but he was unable to work when he had a migraine.

Ted's migraines were fairly frequent—he was missing an average of 2 days of work per month. As is often the case for people with migraines, his boss and the other mechanics weren't convinced that Ted was really suffering all that much. They thought his "migraines" were just an excuse to get out of work early. This added stress didn't help his headaches, and the methysergide prescribed by his doctor didn't seem to be helping much either.

He took sumatriptan to relieve the pain once a migraine had started, but the medication (in oral form) took a few hours to be fully effective. This wasn't fast enough to keep him on the job. Ted genuinely feared losing his job, and he was getting desperate. He was willing to try anything to stop his migraines.

and should be safe for most healthy adults. However, a few side effects are possible. The most significant have been diarrhea and digestive irritation. It is recommended that you reduce your daily dosage level accordingly if you encounter either of these problems.

Individuals with severe heart or kidney disease should not take magnesium (or any other supplement) except on the advice of a physician.

He asked everyone for help. His friends and family members were not at a loss when it came to creative new migraine prevention ideas. It seemed that everyone knew of someone who had gone through an agonizing period of migraine pain before finding some miracle cure or another. Ted tried counseling, he tried meditation, and his cousin made him some herbal tea from the Caribbean. Nothing worked.

Finally, Ted's sister told him about a magazine article she vaguely recalled reading on an in-flight magazine. The article suggested using magnesium to prevent migraines. Ted had nothing to lose. He began taking 600 mg of magnesium each day as a dietary supplement. In the first month, his regular migraine attacks came along as expected. But he kept up with the magnesium. By the second month, for the first time in years, he had only 1 headache. Ted was impressed and continued with the magnesium. With 6 months of this daily routine, Ted was down to 1 fairly mild migraine attack every 2 months. He was missing hardly any days at work, and his confidence was restored.

5-HTP: One Step Away from Serotonin

As we saw in chapter 3, serotonin plays a role in the physiological processes associated with a migraine attack. Research has found that people who are in the middle of a migraine attack have lower serotonin levels than when they are in a headache-free state.[11] Drugs that raise serotonin levels (such as Prozac) or imitate its effects (such as

Imitrex) are widely used for migraines. Another possibility is to stimulate the body into producing more serotonin itself.

On the way to manufacturing serotonin, our bodies produce the substance 5-HTP, or 5-hydroxy tryptophan. Taking 5-HTP supplements might cause the body to produce more serotonin and thus increase overall serotonin levels. While this theory remains unproven, there is some evidence that 5-HTP can help migraines.

Like feverfew, 5-HTP is more widely used in Europe than in the United States. It is most famous as a treatment for depression. (For more information on treatments for depression, see *The Natural Pharmacist Guide to St. John's Wort and Depression*).

What Is the Scientific Evidence for 5-HTP?

There have been a handful of studies on 5-HTP for the prevention of migraines. Three studies compared the use of 5-HTP with the use of conventional migraine medications, and one compared 5-HTP with placebo. Good results were seen in the largest of these studies. (Studies that looked at children are discussed separately below.)

A double-blind study that enrolled 124 people with migraines compared 5-HTP with the standard migraine preventive drug methysergide.[12] According to the results, 5-HTP and methysergide are equally effective at preventing migraine headaches. Seventy-five percent of participants taking methysergide reported at least a 50% reduction in the frequency of attacks or the number of severe attacks. Seventy-one percent of those taking 5-HTP reported likewise. 5-HTP appeared to be more effective in decreasing the intensity and duration of migraine attacks than their frequency.

The side effects associated with the use of methysergide were significantly more serious than those associated with the use of 5-HTP. Fourteen participants using methysergide were withdrawn from the study because of side effects, compared with five using 5-HTP. Side effects experienced by 25% of the methysergide group included nausea, numbness or pain in the legs, insomnia and anxiety, weight gain, impotence, and drowsiness. Side effects experienced by 29% of those taking 5-HTP included abdominal pain, nausea, diarrhea, weight gain, and insomnia.

However, in a smaller double-blind study the conventional antimigraine medication propranolol was shown to be more effective than 5-HTP for the prevention of migraines.[13] The study randomly divided 39 participants into two groups. For 1 month, neither group received treatment (both were given placebo instead). Then the first group received 5-HTP for 4 months, and the second group received propranolol. Propranolol proved more effective both at reducing the duration of attacks and decreasing the need for migraine relief medications.

This study is sometimes incorrectly cited as evidence in favor of 5-HTP. The reason is that both groups improved over the course of the study. However, keep in mind that placebo treatment can be counted on to improve migraine symptoms as well. Since the study was not placebo-controlled, we cannot know whether the improvements noted with 5-HTP were due to its own powers or simply the placebo effect. If 5-HTP had performed as well as propranolol, we might be able to say that since propranolol is known to be better than placebo, 5-HTP must be also. But since propranolol did better than 5-HTP, there really is no legitimate way to use these study results as evidence for the effectiveness of this supplement.

Good results were seen in another double-blind study that compared 5-HTP with the conventional antimigraine medication pizotifen in 80 participants.[14]

A fourth study compared 5-HTP with placebo, but it did not find benefit. In this double-blind randomized study involving 31 participants, half the participants received 400 mg per day of 5-HTP; the other half received placebo.[15] After 2 months—the duration of the study—there was no statistically significant difference between frequency and severity of headaches in the two groups.

However, this study had a serious flaw: The 31 participants all suffered from headaches of some kind or another, but only 16 were actually experiencing migraines. Results for the 16 people with migraines were not analyzed separately, so we don't know if they responded any differently to the treatment than the others. No significant side effects were reported in this study.

The Bottom Line: The best we can really say regarding the use of 5-HTP for the prevention of migraines is that, while initial evidence appears to be promising, its effectiveness remains to be proven.

> **The best we can really say regarding the use of 5-HTP for the prevention of migraines is that, while initial evidence appears to be promising, its effectiveness remains to be proven.**

5-HTP and Children

Several studies have examined the potential effectiveness of 5-HTP for children who suffer from migraines and other forms of headaches. So far, the evidence is again mixed, and more research needs to be done. Most of this research has been carried out in Italy.

One double-blind, crossover, randomized study in Rome examined the effect of daily 5-HTP supplements for 48 elementary and junior high school students who suffered from recurrent headaches and sleep disorders.[16] The researchers of this study were focused on treatments for not only migraines, but rather all headaches that occur in children.

Participants ranged from ages 6 to 16. The 48 students were divided into 2 groups. The daily dosage of L-5-HTP was 4.5 mg for each kg of body weight. One group received 5-HTP for 2 months and then was switched to placebo. The second group received placebo for 2 months, followed by 5-HTP.

Researchers found a statistically significant difference in headache improvement for those taking 5-HTP versus those taking the placebo. There was a 70% reduction in the Headache Index (a measurement tool that recorded headache frequency and intensity) for children taking 5-HTP versus an 11.5% reduction for those taking the placebo. Importantly, there were no reported side effects in this study associated with the use of 5-HTP for the prevention of headaches.

Another Italian study conducted in 1984 found similarly positive results from the use of 5-HTP for children with chronic headaches including, but not exclusively, migraines.[17] However, a similarly designed study in Bologna that enrolled 24 children found no statistical difference between the use of 5-HTP and the use of placebo for migraine prevention in children.[18]

Again, the best that can be said is that while 5-HTP clearly holds promise for children with migraines, more study is necessary.

Nancy's Story

After 20 years of experiencing migraines, Nancy knew how to fend off the well-meaning, free advice of friends, family, and colleagues. She had heard all their folk remedies, from back rubs to warm baths to primordial scream sessions. She had even tried feverfew for several months, but to no avail.

Nancy was appreciative, but enough was enough. She had learned to live with her frequent bouts of pain and suffering—her migraines came about three times per month. She just wanted others to come to the same level of acceptance. Nancy thought of migraines as an inevitable fact in her life—even a part of who she was.

One morning, Nancy rode the bus to work, where she sat behind two older women who were discussing their difficulties with migraines. One of them claimed to have found a great deal of relief from something called 5-HTP. Neither Nancy nor the other woman had ever heard of it, and both were highly skeptical. The woman explained that her sister was a nurse who had learned about it at a health-care workshop.

Warning: Always consult a pediatrician before giving 5-HTP to a child.

Dosage
The typical adult dosage of 5-HTP is 100 to 200 mg taken 3 times per day.

Safety Issues
No significant adverse effects have been reported in clinical trials of 5-HTP. Side effects appear to be limited to

Nancy was intrigued. Although she was tired of getting her hopes up, she did find her migraines pretty tiresome. The next week she asked her pharmacist about 5-HTP.

Her pharmacist knew that some people were using it for migraine prevention, but the evidence supporting it was still very weak. He recommended a dosage of 150 mg per day and told her that he would be very curious to hear about her results.

In the second month of taking 5-HTP, Nancy's average of three migraines was reduced to one, though it was quite severe and very painful. During the following months Nancy's one migraine attack per month decreased in severity, and by the sixth month, she was suffering one mild migraine attack every 6 weeks. One year later, Nancy was thrilled to admit that migraines were no longer an important part of her life.

For every promising new treatment like 5-HTP, there are stories like Nancy's. But only further research can tell us how typical Nancy's experience with 5-HTP was, and how well 5-HTP might work for people with migraines in general.

occasional mild digestive distress and possible allergic reactions.

However, there is one potentially serious concern. In 1998, the U.S. Food and Drug Administration reported detecting a chemical compound in some 5-HTP products known as "peak X." Peak X has a frightening history involving a related supplement: L-tryptophan. Up until about 10 years ago, L-tryptophan was widely used as a sleep aid. The body makes 5-HTP out of L-tryptophan. A certain batch of L-tryptophan supplements caused thousands of cases of a disabling and sometimes fatal blood disorder. Peak X was found to be associated with that disaster.

It is certainly very worrisome to find that the same substance exists in batches of 5-HTP. At press time, there was no other information from the FDA regarding cautions on using specific 5-HTP, but you should pay close attention to media reports that may follow up on this finding.

Safety for young children, pregnant or nursing women, and those with liver or kidney disease has not been established.

Warning: Due to its potential for raising serotonin levels too high, 5-HTP should not be combined with prescription antidepressants.

Acupuncture: A Completely Different Approach

In the world of alternative medicine, acupuncture is commonly believed to be a highly effective treatment for a variety of pain-related ailments, including migraine headaches. However, the scientific evidence for acupuncture is still in its early stages. Evaluating its effectiveness is problematic because of the difficulty of designing anything like a double-blind study.

Acupuncture isn't a pill; it's a treatment administered by a skilled practitioner. In a double-blind study, neither the person receiving nor the person delivering the treatment is supposed to know which is the real medicine and which is the placebo. But there's no way for an acupuncturist not to know whether a treatment is real! As we will see, a kind of double-blind study has been used with acupuncture, but it's not perfect.

What Is the Scientific Evidence for Acupuncture?

In order to approximate a double-blind study, acupuncture researchers use what is called "Sham acupuncture" as placebo. However, it is not fully satisfactory. The method works as follows: First, skilled acupuncturists develop a list of acupuncture points that are generally believed to be helpful in migraine headaches. Next, all the people are treated by technicians who know nothing about acupuncture except how to insert needles. Half of these technicians are given the correct sheet ("Real Acupuncture"), while the others are given a list of points that are not believed to be relevant for migraines ("Sham Acupuncture"). People are divided into two groups, and each group is assigned one group of technicians. The technicians with the "Sham Acupuncture" instructions administer the "placebo" against which the effects of the "Real Acupuncture" will be evaluated. Since neither patients nor technicians know which is which, the treatment is double-blind.

This method has some real problems, however. Properly performed acupuncture is far more sophisticated than what is called "Real Acupuncture" in these studies. Unlike "Real Acupuncture," professional acupuncture is applied in a very individualized way based on specific details of the case—not a list of "migraine points." Also, skilled acupuncturists use many nuances of technique both to precisely locate acupuncture points and to stimulate them, techniques that a barely skilled technician cannot hope to match.

Still, if a study finds that simplified "Real Acupuncture" is more effective than "Sham Acupuncture," it probably means that true acupuncture would be even more effective. However, if the study does not find a difference between the two groups, it does not prove that actual acupuncture applied by an acupuncturist will not work.

There have been a few studies in which acupuncture did seem to help migraine headaches, though not all of them employed the "real" versus "sham" design.

Amazingly, these improvements were found to continue for at least 1 year following the termination of acupuncture treatment. This suggests that acupuncture is doing more than just relieving symptoms.

One randomized, controlled study involving 30 participants with migraines found that acupuncture could reduce both the frequency and intensity of migraine attacks.[19] Amazingly, these improvements were found to continue for at least 1 year following the termination of acupuncture treatment. This is particularly exciting because it suggests that acupuncture is doing more than just relieving symptoms.

The 30 participants were divided into two groups. One group received a "real" acupuncture treatment, while the other received a "sham" acupuncture treatment. Those who received "real" acupuncture reported significant reductions in both the intensity and frequency of their migraine attacks, compared with those who received the "sham" treatment. There was also a 38% reduction in the use of migraine medications among those receiving the "real" treatment. This remained true in follow-ups occurring 4 months and 1 year after the completion of the treatment.

In another study, this time with no controls, it was found that 5 acupuncture treatments given to 39 people with migraines over a 1-month period initially reduced the frequency of migraines for 92% of participants. Six months later, 54% of the participants had relapsed to their pre-acupuncture state.[20] As the author acknowledges, however, there is very little we can conclude from this finding, since there's no way to know how much the benefits were influenced by the placebo effect.

How Much Acupuncture Will I Need?

Acupuncture is generally administered at the rate of once or twice a week. There is not enough information at this time to recommend any particular length of treatment. Most acupuncturists would probably agree that the longer you've had migraines, the longer it might take for acupuncture to change the pattern of your headaches. In real life, acupuncture is more of a craft than a science. Some practitioners simply seem to be far more skilled than others.

> **In real life, acupuncture is more of a craft than a science. Some practitioners simply seem to be far more skilled than others.**

It is worth taking the time to identify a highly skilled acupuncturist, rather than picking one at random out of the phone book. Acupuncturists should have completed 2 to 3 years of full-time training and be certified by the National Commission for the Certification of Acupuncturists (NCCA). In many states, they can be given one of the following titles: Certified Acupuncturist, Licensed Acupuncturist, or Registered Acupuncturist. Chiropractors (DCs) and medical physicians (MDs) are generally permitted to practice acupuncture with much less training, ranging from no training at all to a 3-month course.

Basic qualifications are much easier to ascertain than the acupuncturist's skill. I recommend getting informed referrals from people who have received acupuncture, especially if they have enough experience with it to have tried more than one practitioner. A health-care practitioner who has referred many people for acupuncture may also be able to give you a good recommendation. Finally, there are many schools or systems of acupuncture, and some may work better for you than others.

Safety Issues

Acupuncture is quite safe. As long as you make sure that the acupuncturist has the basic qualifications, the worst side effects you are likely to experience are slight bleeding on the skin where a needle is placed, temporary discomfort, and an occasional bruise. It's not unusual for the headache pain to get temporarily worse before it gets better. Your acupuncturist can give you an idea of what kind of changes to expect.

The acupuncturist should use disposable needles to dispense with the risk of communicating HIV or hepatitis. Rare but more severe side effects include puncture of the lung or other internal organs, and severe bleeding (mostly in people who are taking blood thinners). An acupuncturist is specifically trained to avoid these disasters. However, those taking blood thinners such as Coumadin (warfarin) should probably not try acupuncture at all, due to the increased risk of bleeding complications.

An additional problem with acupuncture is its cost. Acupuncture typically costs from $40 to $100 per session, making it more expensive than the other treatments discussed in this book. (Some health insurance plans cover acupuncture.) However, if it produces a long-lasting effect that persists beyond the end of treatment, as the above-mentioned study suggests, you might feel that it's worth it.

Fish Oil: Preventing Migraines While Improving Your Health

Our grandparents used to take cod-liver oil as a health tonic, and today fish oil is thought to be good for us in several ways. (For more information on the possible health benefits of fish oil, see *The Natural Pharmacist: Your Complete Guide to Vitamins and Supplements*.) Because ingesting fish oil tends to decrease platelet aggregation, it has been speculated that it might be useful in preventing migraines. Platelet aggregation causes the release of serotonin, which may be associated with the onset of a migraine attack.[21]

Very small, controlled studies have suggested that high dosages of fish oil may help prevent migraines.

Very small, controlled studies have suggested that high dosages of fish oil may help prevent migraines.[22,23] However, this research is extremely preliminary.

Dosage

A typical dosage is 6 to 9 g (taken in 1-g capsules) of fish oil daily. Cod-liver oil may not be the best choice, however (see below). Many other types are available.

Safety Issues

Cod-liver oil may not be the best form of fish oil because it contains so much vitamin D and A, vitamins that can become toxic when taken to excess. Pregnant women in particular must not take overdoses of vitamin A. Safer sources include oil from salmon, mackerel, and herring.

Fish oil can modestly raise low-density lipoproteins in the blood (also known as "bad" cholesterol), although this effect usually goes away after some months of continuous ingestion. Fish oil should be sold combined with vitamin E to prevent its being oxidized into less healthful forms.

Warning: Fish oil should not be combined with blood thinners such as aspirin or Coumadin (warfarin) except under the supervision of a physician.

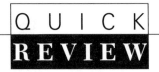

QUICK REVIEW

- Beyond the use of feverfew, a number of other alternative medical therapies have shown some promise for preventing migraines.

- Small double-blind trials suggest that magnesium supplements may reduce the frequency of migraines. A typical daily dosage is 360 to 600 mg. Magnesium in this dosage is safe for healthy adults, although it can occasionally cause mild diarrhea and digestive irritation.

- Some evidence also suggests that the supplement 5-HTP may reduce the frequency and intensity of migraine attacks. A typical adult dosage is 100 to 200 mg taken 3 times per day.

- Highly preliminary studies suggest that acupuncture may reduce the severity and frequency of migraines. The most exciting possibility is that the benefits may last long after treatment is stopped. However, much more research is necessary.

- Fish oil may also help prevent migraines.

Other Types of Headaches

A s we have seen, the herb feverfew appears to reduce the frequency and severity of migraine headaches. However, feverfew probably only works for migraines, and migraines aren't the only kind of headache. This chapter briefly describes the other common headache types, how to distinguish them from migraines, and how to treat them. There are three principal types of nonmigraine headaches: tension, sinus, and TMJ/dental headaches.

Tension head-aches are the most common form of headache.

Tension Headaches

Tension headaches are the most common form of headache. They account for nearly 90% of all headaches. Tension headaches feel like a pressing pain around the circumference of your skull, a bandlike pain wrapping your entire head. One woman who suffered from tension headaches for many years compared her pain to "a vice clamping down on my head while the muscles in the back of my neck are slowly pulled out at their roots." This vivid description should be familiar to anyone who has ever had to endure a serious bout of tension headaches.

Tension headaches feel like a pressing pain around the circumference of your skull, a band-like pain wrapping your entire head.

As with migraine headaches, women suffer in greater numbers than men. An estimated 88% of women experience tension headaches at some point in their lives, compared to an estimated 69% of men. Most people are between 20 and 40 years of age when they first begin to experience them.

In the past, tension headaches have not always been taken as seriously as they deserve. This is because the pain is often less severe and they are seen more as a nuisance than potentially disabling. In recent years, however, researchers and doctors are increasingly recognizing that tension headaches—especially chronic ones—are a serious health problem.

A major Ohio University study has compared tension headaches with other chronic diseases (such as chronic fatigue syndrome and arthritis), in terms of the pain and disruption they cause. The study's findings were presented to the annual meeting of the American Association for the Study of Headache in June 1998. It was found that 2 to 3% of all Americans suffer from chronic tension headaches, and two-thirds of those have pain almost every day. More than 70% have trouble with sleeping, fatigue, anxiety, and stress due to their headaches. In a survey of

Helpful Clues to Distinguish a Migraine from a Tension Headache

Although there is no guaranteed way of distinguishing between a tension headache and a migraine, the following is a list of the most important and common distinguishing features.

Migraine Headache	Tension Headache
Severe, throbbing, pulsating pain focused in one area, often above or behind one eye.	Dull, aching, bandlike pain wrapping around the whole head and throughout the head.
Aggravated by physical activity.	Not aggravated by physical activity.
Associated with nausea/ vomiting; sensitivity to light, sound, and odors; and possibly preceded by aura.	No nausea/vomiting; sensitivity to light, sound, and odors; or aura.

245 people suffering from chronic tension headaches, 72% reported having missed school or work an average of 3.5 times in the previous 6 months. Researchers noted, "These headaches are disrupting lives as much or more than other chronic diseases."

Because they are so common, tension headaches have had several different names, including "tension-type headache," "muscle tension headache," "muscle contraction headache," "stress headache," and "ordinary headache." As we might guess from this variety of names, the medical practice of categorizing headaches is still evolving and imperfect. Diagnosing a tension headache is not an exact science. In chapter 2, we saw that it is very important for people with migraine headaches to be able to communicate well with their doctors. This is equally true for tension headaches. The nature of the pain associated with tension headaches varies widely.

Intensity of Pain

Most people who suffer from tension headaches describe the pain as mild to moderate. Usually, the pain is annoying and distracting, but manageable. Nonetheless, tension headaches can cause people to miss work or school. As we saw above in the woman's vivid description of her pain, a tension headache can indeed be uncomfortably intense. It is only "moderate" when compared to the blinding pain of a severe migraine.

In general, tension headaches are milder than the worst migraines, but the distinction isn't always so clear in real life. Migraines can be relatively mild, and tension headaches can be painful enough to disrupt your life. To correctly diagnose your headache, you and your doctor will need to look at the overall pattern of all your symptoms.

Duration of Tension Headaches

Other types of headache may be more intense, but tension headaches have a wicked staying power. One way to distinguish a tension headache from a migraine is by the duration of the attack. A typical migraine lasts for 3 to 12 hours, while most tension headaches last for a shorter period of 2 to 3 hours. However, tension headaches can occur as often as daily and can last for days at a time. Indeed, some people report that their pain ebbs and surges but never truly goes away at all.

Tension headaches, for some reason, most often begin in the early morning and early evening. The onset of a tension headache may be either gradual or relatively sudden. There is no aura.

Frequency of Tension Headaches

People who suffer from tension headaches are categorized according to the frequency of their headaches. *Episodic* sufferers have a tension headache on less than 15 days each month. *Chronic* tension headache occurs on 15 or more days each month—a chronic tension headache is an ordinary part of everyday life for the person experiencing the headache. In the long term, such chronic pain can become a serious health problem. By comparison, migraines rarely occur more often than once or twice a week, although they are usually more severe.

Location of Pain

The pain of a tension headache is generally located in your forehead and temples, or down the back of your head, neck, and shoulders. It often feels like a band wrapping tightly around your head. The pain may appear on both sides of your head, or just one. In about half of all tension headache attacks, the pain shifts from one location to another. The bandlike pressure is the key symptom of a tension headache. Migraines or other types of headaches rarely feature this bandlike pressure.

Type of Pain

Most people with tension headaches describe the pain as a steady, dull, nonpulsating ache. People with tension headaches report a significant variety of experiences.

All tension headaches generally begin with a dull band of pain around the circumference of the head. For some, the pain grows in intensity before leveling off and remaining an annoying presence for up to 12 hours. For others, the pain grows in intensity to beyond a mere annoyance and briefly disrupts their day before subsiding partially or completely. This ache is generally quite mild at the outset of a tension headache, but it gradually builds.

As we've seen, it isn't always easy to distinguish the pain of a migraine headache from that of a tension headache. Usually, though, a tension headache involves a pressurelike sensation wrapping the entire head rather than the pulsating, throbbing, more localized pain of a migraine.

Tension Headache Symptoms Other Than Head Pain

As with a migraine headache, a tension headache has important symptoms aside from the immediate head pain. Your scalp may be so tender during a headache that it hurts to comb your hair or even wear a hat. This tenderness at the site of your headache can persist for several days following a tension headache. Another common symptom of a tension headache is tightness in the neck or jaw.

The most common treatments for tension headaches are over-the-counter analgesics such as aspirin, acetaminophen (Tylenol), and ibuprofen.

Conventional Treatment of Tension Headaches

The most common treatment for the occasional tension headache is an over-the-counter analgesic such as aspirin, acetaminophen (Tylenol), and ibuprofen. These medicines can be quite effective in relieving the mild pain of a tension headache. Chronic tension headaches, on the other hand, usually require stronger medication. Doctors often prescribe antidepres-

Bob's Story

Bob first began to notice his headaches after he turned 23. At first, he didn't think of them as actual headaches. They felt more like a light but steady band of pressure wrapped around his head. For Bob, this was annoying but not particularly painful.

Then, as the months passed, he began to notice that he was having more and more episodes of this wrapping sensation. With each new round, the pressure seemed to increase. But the headaches didn't come very often, and Bob still wasn't worried. At one point, during a work-required routine physical examination, a doctor asked him whether he had headaches. Because Bob didn't think his mild, occasional headaches were worth mentioning, he didn't say anything.

However, within only 3 months of this medical exam, Bob's headaches suddenly began to get worse, until he was having two to three episodes a week of fairly painful tension headaches. He began to develop a stomachache from all the aspirin he was taking and started missing days at work, losing sleep, and developing a general feeling of anxiety.

At this point, his doctor became involved. He diagnosed Bob as having chronic tension headaches and placed him on antidepressants. The antidepressants proved effective in alleviating his insomnia, lowering his anxiety level, and cutting down on the frequency of his headaches.

sants, which may relieve pain for reasons that are not entirely understood.[1,2] Muscle relaxant drugs are also occasionally helpful, although they tend to cause too much drowsiness to be very useful.

Because chronic tension headaches tend to occur on a long-term basis, it is important to avoid the use of habit-forming drugs, such as tranquilizers and narcotic pain relievers.

Alternative treatments that might be helpful for tension headaches include massage, acupuncture, chiropractic, and the herb kava. (For more information on kava, see *The Natural Pharmacist Guide to Kava and Anxiety*.)

Sinus Headaches

To see if you have a true sinus headache, bend forward. If the pain in your forehead and face intensifies significantly, you probably have a sinus headache.

Sinus headaches are among the most painful headaches you can experience. Your sinuses are tunnels beneath the layers of bone that form a cavity behind your forehead, the bridge of your nose, and your cheekbones. These sinus tunnels have walls lined with mucus-secreting membranes.

When sinus passages become blocked by an infection or allergy, the mucous can build up. As mucus accumulates, the sinus tissue tends to swell. This creates pressure and eventually pain as the sinus linings push against nerve endings in the sinuses. The swelling and inflammation of the sinus can also cause the blood vessels in the mucus membranes to expand. This dilation of the blood vessels adds a vascular element to your already painful sinus headache.

As with any headache, a proper diagnosis of your sinus headache is the first step in treating it. The nature of the pain associated with sinus headaches varies widely.

Helpful Clues to Distinguish a Migraine from a Sinus Headache

The easiest way to distinguish between sinus and migraine headaches is to bend forward. If the pain in your forehead and face intensifies significantly, you probably have a sinus headache. Some other distinctions are as follows:

Migraine Headache	Sinus Headache
Often one-sided.	One-sided or two-sided.
Above or behind one eye.	Pain either between the eyebrows, in the forehead, behind the cheekbones, or behind the eyes.
Throbbing pain that peaks and then decreases.	
Associated with nausea/vomiting; sensitivity to light, sound, and odors; and possibly preceded by aura.	Gnawing, dull, aching pain that gradually increases over time.
	Movement of head forward and back (as if bowing) intensifies pain.
	Often associated with dizziness, nasal stuffiness.

Intensity of Pain

The intensity of pain experienced by people with sinus headaches ranges from moderate to severe or even debilitating. A full sinus headache episode involves severe, debilitating pain in the sinus area of the head. A person with headaches often experiences nasal discharge, ear sensations (or fullness), and facial swelling as the pain grows in intensity. Any movement of the head will shoot searing waves of pain through the sinus area. This is one of the most debilitating types of headache. As with migraines, the pain is often intense enough to force someone to lie down.

However, unlike a migraine, which tends to peak and then diminish slowly, a sinus headache gradually becomes more painful over the course of the headache episode. For some, the attack simply comes to a close; for others, the pain responds well to medication.

> **Unlike a migraine, which tends to peak and then diminish slowly, a sinus headache gradually becomes more painful over the course of the headache episode.**

Duration of Sinus Headache

Sinus headaches generally last from 1 to 24 hours. However, some sinus episodes have been known to last as long as several weeks. Some sinus headaches can subside on their own without medication.

Frequency of Sinus Headaches

There is no regular pattern of frequency for sinus headaches.

Location of Pain

The location of migraine and sinus headaches can be very similar. Your sinuses are like tunnels drilled within the layers of bone beneath your forehead, the bridge of your nose, and your cheekbones. These tunnels form three sinus groups. The precise location of the pain depends on which sinus group is affected. Generally, the pain will either be between your eyebrows, behind the eyes, above your eyebrows, or behind your cheekbones. A sinus headache can involve two, or even all three, sinus groups.

Type of Pain

Sinus headache pain is most often described as a deep, dull, gnawing ache. The onset of a sinus headache tends to be gradual. Where migraine pain is usually described as throbbing or pulsating, sinus headache pain is constant and steady. The pain is often described as more severe than that of a migraine. At its worst, the sinus headache can feel like an ice pick planted squarely between your eyes. The pain of a sinus headache grows more intense with head movement, and the affected sinus area is often tender to the touch.

Sinus Headache
Symptoms Other Than Head Pain

With a sinus headache, one or both of your temples may feel swollen. You may develop coldlike symptoms such as a low-grade fever, teary eyes, sneezing, and discharge from the nose or the back of the throat. Additionally, you may temporarily lose your sense of smell, and the headache pain may radiate down to your teeth.

Conventional Treatment of Sinus Headaches

Because a sinus headache is caused by the buildup of mucus in your sinus cavities, the first order of business in treating a sinus headache is to clear your sinus passageways and treat the infection, if one is present. There are three basic approaches within conventional medicine to open clogged sinus passages and to attack bacterial infection:

1. Decongestants and the mucus-loosening medication guaifenesin (Humabid) are used to help unblock the sinus passageways.

2. Antihistamines or, in severe cases, corticosteroids, may be prescribed to reduce allergy-related swelling.

3. Antibiotics may be prescribed to attack the offending sinus infection.

Some people with chronic sinus infections may eventually need microsurgery to widen their sinus passages.

The most commonly used alternative treatment for sinus headaches is identifying and eliminating food allergens (such as milk). Acupuncture may be helpful as well.

TMJ/Dental Headaches

The temporomandibular joint (TMJ) is the hinge that attaches your lower jaw, or mandible, with your skull, allow-

A TMJ/dental headache is caused by spasm and fatigue in the muscles surrounding the temporomandibular joint.

ing you to open and close your mouth. If you place a finger at the base of each ear as you chew, you can feel the TMJ working. This important facial joint extends all the way to your temple.

The TMJ is a workhorse; on a typical day, we open and close our jaws over 2,000 times. But the TMJ is vulnerable to stress and fatigue. Dental problems such as misalignment can force the jaw muscles and TMJ to work harder than they should.

A TMJ/dental headache is caused by spasm and fatigue in the muscles surrounding this joint. This is because the muscles that work the TMJ extend all the way up to the

Helpful Clues to Distinguish a Migraine from a TMJ/Dental Headache

It is important to remember that the following descriptions provide only general criteria of the differences between TMJ headaches and migraines.

Migraine Headache	TMJ/Dental Headache
Often one-sided.	Sides of head.
Above or behind one eye.	Tenderness in jaw area.
Throbbing pain.	Dull pain located near the jaw joint or spread throughout the head.
Often associated with nausea/vomiting; sensitivity to light, sounds, and odors; and may be preceded by aura.	Often accompanied by clicking or "thunking" sound in jaw when opening/closing mouth.

temples. The nature of the pain associated with TMJ headaches varies widely.

Intensity of Pain

The intensity of pain associated with a TMJ/dental headache is usually mild to moderate. In general, TMJ/dental headaches are less intensely painful than migraines and the other headaches described in this chapter. However, the pain may ultimately wear you down by its perpetual presence.

For example, Joe is a 32-year-old carpenter who suffers from TMJ headaches. He describes his pain as a dull, gnawing, ever-present pain in the region of his jaw. The pain is a constant companion throughout the day and can be only slightly deadened by over-the-counter pain relievers. It hurts most when he chews.

Duration of TMJ/Dental Headaches

TMJ/dental headaches tend to cause simmering, continuous discomfort.

Frequency of TMJ/Dental Headaches

TMJ/dental headaches can range in frequency from occasional to constant. Eating or yawning may trigger a headache.

The pain of a TMJ/dental headache tends to be located near the jaw joint, but it may spread to wrap around the head as well.

Location of Pain

The pain of a TMJ/dental headache tends to be located near the jaw joint, but it may spread to wrap around the head as well.

Type of Pain

Most people with TMJ/dental headaches describe their pain as a dull, steady pressure. Like tension headaches, TMJ/dental headaches are often described as having a clamping, bandlike pressure. The pain tends to intensify when you chew, and can give you the sensation of muscle spasms in the area of the jaw.

TMJ/Dental Headache Symptoms Other Than Head Pain

TMJ/dental headaches are often accompanied by a tenderness around your jaw, within your mouth, and in the area where your jaw meets your skull. Unusual popping, clicking, or cracking sounds in the jaw may also occur.

Treatment for TMJ/Dental Headaches

Because the teeth, temporomandibular joints, and chewing muscles can all play a role, the treatment for TMJ/dental headaches can vary. Standard treatment includes anti-inflammatory drugs, muscle relaxants, and the use of an orthotic, a special dental splint worn over the teeth to keep the jaw from closing fully. Surgery is tried in some cases. Alternative treatments for TMJ/dental headaches include deep-tissue massage, cranial-sacral osteopathy, and acupuncture.

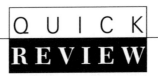

QUICK REVIEW

- Feverfew is probably only effective for migraine headaches. However, you can have more than one type of headache at once.

- Tension headaches are the most common type of headache. Caused by muscle tension, they typically feel like a dull, bandlike pain over the whole head.

- Sinus headaches consist of inflammation or pressure in the sinuses. The pain can be in the forehead, behind the cheekbones, or behind or between the eyes. When you bow your head forward, the pain usually increases.

- TMJ/dental headaches can cause constant, nagging, low-level pain, often accompanied by a "click" or "thunk" in the jaw.

Putting It All Together

For your easy reference, this chapter contains a brief summary of key information contained in this book. Please refer to earlier chapters for more comprehensive information, including a detailed discussion of safety issues.

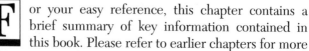

Migraine Headaches

Headache can be an indicator of certain more serious medical conditions. See a physician to make sure your headaches *are* migraines before you use the treatments described in this book.

Migraine headaches can be difficult to diagnose. Although there is a "classic" pattern of migraine symptoms, most people's migraines vary from this pattern. It's important that you and your doctor communicate well about your headaches so that a proper diagnosis can be made.

There are two basic kinds of migraine treatment: relief and prevention. Pain relief medications, such as sumatriptan, stop the pain of a headache once it's begun, while migraine prevention treatments, such as feverfew, work to reduce the frequency of migraines or eliminate them altogether. You may wish to have your physician prescribe a conventional medication, such as sumatriptan, for migraine relief, even while you take feverfew for prevention.

Feverfew and Migraines

In England, feverfew has been used as a folk remedy for the prevention of migraines for many centuries. Available research suggests that regular use of feverfew can reduce the frequency and intensity of migraines.

The primary advantage of feverfew over conventional medications is that it seems to be virtually free of side effects. The standard dosage is 80 to 100 mg per day of dried feverfew leaves in capsule form. Feverfew extracts may not be effective.

It was once thought that the active ingredient in feverfew was parthenolide, but a recent study has called this into question. Still, when purchasing powdered feverfew leaf, it may be worthwhile to choose products known to contain from 0.2 to 0.66% parthenolide in order to match the product used in the studies with positive results.

If you chew feverfew leaf from your garden you may develop mouth sores, tongue inflammation, and stomach distress. Feverfew capsules don't seem to cause this problem.

Based on the known effects of feverfew, it is possible that the herb may interact with drugs that "thin" the blood, such as Coumadin (warfarin), heparin, or aspirin. I suggest avoiding such combinations except on the advice of a physician.

We don't know if feverfew is safe for young children, pregnant or nursing mothers, or those with severe liver or kidney disease.

Other Natural Treatments for Migraines

Besides feverfew, other nondrug treatments, such as **magnesium, 5-HTP, acupuncture,** and **fish oil,** may be helpful for preventing migraines. Please see chapter 8 for additional information regarding the safety of these treatments and the evidence that they are effective. The standard dosage of magnesium is 350 to 600 mg daily. The typical adult dosage of 5-HTP is 100 to 200 mg 3 times a day. A typical dosage of fish oil is three to six 1-gram capsules daily. Make sure to find a qualified acupuncturist, as not all practitioners are equally skillful.

Notes

Introduction

1. Silberstein S, et al. Migraine: Diagnosis and treatment. In: Dalessio D, Silberstein D, eds. Wolff's headache and other head pain, 6th Ed. New York: Oxford University Press, 136–139, 1993.

2. Silberstein S, et al., 1993.

3. Raskin N. Migraine and cluster headache syndrome. In: Fauci A, Braunwald E, Isselbacher K, Wilson J, Martin J, Kasper D, Hauser S, Longo D, eds. Harrison's internal medicine, New York: McGraw Hill, 2307–2311, 1998.

Chapter One

1. Castleman M. The healing herbs. Emmaus, PA: Rodale Press, 173–176, 1991.

2. Castleman M, 1991.

Chapter Two

1. Goadsby P, et al. Diagnosis and management of migraine. *Br Med J* 312: 1278–1283, 1996.

2. Brukner H. Update on migraine headaches. http://uhs.bsd.uchicago.edu/uhs/topics/migraine.html

3. Blau J. Migraine prodromes separated from the aura. *Br Med J* 281: 658–660, 1980.

4. Brukner H. Update on migraine headaches. http://uhs.bsd
.uchicago.edu/uhs/topics/migraine.html

Chapter Three

1. Lance J. The pathophysiology of migraine. In: Dalessio D,
Silberstein S, eds. Wolff's headache and other head pain, 6th
Ed. New York: Oxford University Press, 59–96, 1993.

2. Welch K. Migraine: A biobehavioral disorder. *Arch Neurol*
44: 323, 1987.

3. Olesen J. Cerebral and extracranial circulatory disturbances
in migraine: Pathophysiological implications. *Cerebrovasc
Brain Metab* Rev 3:1, 1991.

4. Woods R, et al. Brief report: Bilateral spreading cerebral
hypoperfusion during spontaneous migraine headache.
N Engl J Med 331: 1689, 1995.

5. Lance J, et al., 1993.

6. Rapoport A, et al. Headache disorders: a management guide
for practitioners. Philadelphia: WB Saunders, 1996.

7. Rapoport A, et al., 1996.

8. Rapoport A, et al., 1996.

9. Ferrari M, et al. Neuroexcitatory plasma amino acids are elevated in migraine. *Neurology* 40: 1582–1586, 1990.

Chapter Four

1. Rapoport A, et al. Headache disorders: a management guide
for practitioners. Philadelphia: WB Saunders, 1996.

2. Scheftell F, et al. Subcutaneous sumatriptan in a clinical setting: The first 100 consecutive patients with acute migraine
in a tertiary care center. *Headache* 34: 67, 1994.

3. Rapoport A, et al., 1996.

4. Scheftell F, et al., 1994.

5. American Council on Headache Education (ACHE). Migraine: the complete guide. New York: Dell Publishing,
1994.

6. Ziegler D, The treatment of migraine. In Dalessio D, ed. Wolff's headache and other head pain, 5th Ed. New York: Oxford University Press, 87–111, 1987.

7. Rapoport A, et al., 1996.

8. Rapoport A, et al., 1996.

9. Brooks P, et al. Nonsteroidal anti-inflammatory drugs—differences and similarities. *N Engl J Med* 324: 1716–1725, 1991.

10. Rapoport A, et al., 1996.

11. Henry P, et al. Ergotamine- and analgesic-induced headaches. In: Rose C, ed. *Migraine.* London, 197–205, 1985.

12. Peters B, et al. Comparison of 650 mg aspirin and 1000 mg acetaminophen with each other, and with placebo in moderately severe headache. *Am J Med* 76: 36–42, 1983.

13. Murray W, et al. Evaluation of aspirin in treatment of headache. *Clin Pharmacol Ther* 5: 21–25, 1964.

14. Ryan R. A study of Midrin in the symptomatic relief of migraine headache. *Headache* 14: 33–42, 1974.

15. Yuill G, et al. A double-blind crossover trial of isometheptene mucate compound and ergotamine in migraine. *Br J Clin Pract* 26: 76–79, 1972.

16. Rapoport A, et al., 1996.

17. Saper J. Chronic opioid Rx for non-malignant pain? *Top Pain Management* 5: 45, 1990.

18. Boyle R, et al. A correlation between severity of migraine and delayed emptying measured by an epigastric impedance method. *Br J Clin Pharmacol* 30: 405–409, 1990.

19. Tfelt-Hansen P, et al. A double-blind study of metoclopramide in the treatment of migraine attacks. *J Neurol Neurosurg Psychiatry* 43: 369–371, 1980.

20. Raskin N. Migraine and cluster headache syndrome. In: Fauci A, Braunwald E, Isselbacher K, Wilson J, Martin J, Kasper D, Hauser S, Longo D, eds. Harrison's internal medicine, New York: McGraw Hill, 2307–2311, 1998.

21. Andersson K., et al. Beta-adrenoceptor blockers and calcium antagonists in the prophylaxis and treatment of migraine. *Drugs* 39: 355–373, 1990.

22. Curran D, et al. Clinical trial of methysergide and other preparations in the management of migraine. *J Neurol Neurosurg Psychiatry* 27: 463–469, 1964.

23. Silberstein S, et al. Migraine: Diagnosis and treatment. In: Dalessio D, Silberstein D, eds. Wolff's headache and other head pain, 6th Ed. New York: Oxford University Press, 136–139, 1993.

24. Rapoport A, et al. Headache disorders: a management guide for practitioners. Philadelphia: WB Saunders, 1996.

25. Andersson K, et al., 1990.

26. Rapoport A, et al., 1996.

27. Silberstein S, et al., 1993.

28. Rapoport A, et al., 1996.

Chapter Five

1. Johnson E, et al. Efficacy of feverfew as prophylactic treatment of migraine. *Br Med J* 291: 569–573, 1985.

2. Murphy J, et al. Randomized double-blind placebo-controlled trial of feverfew in migraine prevention. *Lancet* 8604: 189–192, 1988.

3. Heptinstall S, et al. Extracts of feverfew inhibit granule secretion in blood platelets and polymorphonuclear leucocytes. *Lancet* 8437: 1071–1074, 1985.

4. Groenewegen W, et al. Compounds extracted from feverfew that have anti-secretory activity contain a butyrolactone unit. *J Pharm Pharmacol* 39: 709–712, 1987.

5. Collier H, et al. Extract of feverfew inhibits prostaglandin biosynthesis. *Lancet* ii: 922–923, 1980.

6. Makheja A, et al. A platelet phospholipase inhibitor from the medicinal herb feverfew. *Prostaglandins Leukotr Med* 8: 653–660, 1982.

7. De Weerdt C, et al. Randomized double-blind placebo-controlled crossover trial of a feverfew preparation. *Phytomedicine* 3: 225–230, 1996.

8. Palevitch D, et al. Feverfew as a prophylactic treatment for migraine: a double-blind placebo-controlled study. *Phytother Res* 11: 508–511, 1997.

9. Palevitch D, et al., 1997.

10. Williams C, et al. A biologically active lipophilic flavonol from *Tanacetum parthenium*. *Phytochemistry* 38: 267–270, 1995.

11. Tyler V. Herbs of choice. New York: Pharmaceutical Production Press, 1994.

Chapter Seven

1. Murphy J, et al. Randomized double-blind placebo-controlled trial of feverfew in migraine prevention. *Lancet* 8604: 189–192, 1988.

2. Johnson E, et al. Efficacy of feverfew as prophylactic treatment of migraine. *Br Med J* 291: 569–573, 1985.

3. Baldwin C. What pharmacists should know about feverfew. *Pharm J* 239: 237–238, 1987.

4. Anderson D, et al. Chromosomal aberrations and sister chromatid exchanges in lymphocytes and urine mutagenicity of migraine patients: a comparison of chronic feverfew users and matched non-users. *Hum Toxicol* 7: 145–152, 1988.

5. ESCOP Monographs Fascicule II. Tanaceti parhenii herba/folium P3. Exeter, UK: European Commission on Phytotherapy, 1996.

Chapter Eight

1. Mazzotta G, et al. Electromyographical ischemic test and intracellular and extracellular magnesium concentration in migraine and tension type headache patients. *Headache* 36: 357–361, 1996.

2. Ramadan N, et al. Low brain magnesium in migraine. *Headache* 29: 590–593, 1989.

3. Ramadan N, et al., 1989.

4. Swanson D. Migraine and magnesium: eleven neglected connections. *Perspect Biol Med* 31: 526–561, 1988.

5. Peikert A, et al. Prophylaxis of migraine with oral magnesium: results from a prospective, multi-center, placebo-controlled and double-blind randomized study. *Cephalagia* 16: 257–263, 1996.

6. Taubert K. Magnesium in migraine: results of a multicenter pilot study [Abstract]. *Only Fortschr Med* 112(24): 328–30, 1994.

7. Facchinetti F, et al. Magnesium prophylaxis of menstrual migraine: effects on intracellular magnesium. *Headache* 31: 298–301, 1991.

8. Facchinetti F, et al., 1991.

9. Pfaffenrath V, et al. Magnesium in the prophylaxis of migraine: a double-blind placebo-controlled study. *Cephalagia* 16: 436–440, 1996.

10. Gaby AR. Research review. *Nutrition & Healing,* 1997.

11. Titus F, et al. 5-Hydroxytryptophan versus methysergide in the prophylaxis of migraine: randomized clinical trial. *Eur Neurol* 25: 327–329, 1986.

12. Titus F, et al., 1986.

13. Maissen C, et al. Comparison of the effect of 5-hydroxytryptophan and propranolol in the interval treatment of migraine. *Med Wochenschr* 121: 1585–1590, 1991.

14. Bono G, et al. Serotonin precursors in migraine prophylaxis. *Adv Neurol* 33: 357–363, 1982.

15. De Benedittis G, et al. Serotonin precursors in chronic primary headache: a double-blind crossover study with L-5-hydroxytryptophan versus placebo. *J Neurosurg Sci* 29: 239–248, 1985.

16. De Giorgis G, et al. Headache in association with sleep disorders in children: a psychodiagnostic evaluation. *Drugs Exp Clin Res* 13: 425–433, 1987.

17. Longo G, et al. Treatment of essential headache in developmental age with 5-hydroxytryptophan: crossover double-blind study versus placebo. *Pediatr Med Chir* 6: 241–245, 1984.

18. Santucci M, et al. L-5-Hydroxytryptophan versus placebo in childhood migraine prophylaxis: a double-blind crossover study. *Cephalagia* 6: 155–157, 1986.

19. Vincent C. A controlled trial of the treatment of migraine by acupuncture. *Clin J Pain* 5: 305–312, 1989.

20. Laitinen J. Acupuncture for migraine prophylaxis: a prospective clinical study with six month's follow-up. *Am J Chin Med* 3: 271–274, 1975.

21. Woodcock B, et al. Beneficial effect of fish oil on blood viscosity in peripheral vascular disease. *Br Med J* 288: 592–594, 1984.

22. Glueck C, et al. Amelioration of severe migraine with omega-3 fatty acids: a double-blind placebo-controlled clinical trial [Abstract]. *Am J Clin Nutr* 43: 710, 1986.

23. McCarren T, et al. Amelioration of severe migraine by fish oil (w-3) fatty acids [Abstract]. *Am J Clin Nutr* 41: 874a, 1985.

Chapter Nine

1. Diamond S. Tension-type headaches. In: Dalessio D, Silberstein S, eds. Wolff's headache and other head pain, 6th Ed. New York: Oxford University Press, 235–261, 1993.

2. Ravaris C, et al. Phenelzine and amitriptyline in treatment of depression: a comparison of present and past studies. *Arch Gen Psychiatry* 37: 1057–1080, 1980.

Index

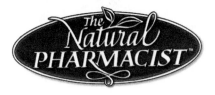

About the Author

David Baronov has been a science and medical writer for the past 10 years. He currently works with Bastyr University's Research Institute in the Pacific Northwest, designing research projects that evaluate the efficacy of various natural medicine treatments. He lives in Seattle, Washington, with his wife, Maria, and son, Andre.

About the Series Editors

Steven Bratman, M.D., medical director of Prima Health, has many years of experience in the alternative medicine field. A graduate of the University of California at Davis, Medical School, he has also trained in herbology, nutrition, Chinese medicine, and other alternative therapies, and has worked closely with a wide variety of alternative practitioners. He is the author of *The Natural Pharmacist: Your Complete Guide to Herbs* (Prima), *The Natural Pharmacist: Your Complete Guide to Illnesses and Their Natural Remedies* (Prima), *The Natural Pharmacist Guide to St. John's Wort and Depression* (Prima), *The Alternative Medicine Ratings Guide* (Prima), and *The Alternative Medicine Sourcebook* (Lowell House).

David J. Kroll, Ph.D., is a professor of pharmacology and toxicology at the University of Colorado School of Pharmacy and a consultant for pharmacists, physicians, and alternative practitioners on the indications and cautions for herbal medicine use. A graduate of both the University of Florida and the Philadelphia College of Pharmacy and Science, Dr. Kroll has lectured widely and has published articles in a number of medical journals, abstracts, and newsletters.